In Sickness and in Health

Arthur C. Blais

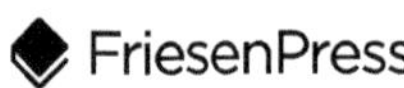

One Printers Way
Altona, MB R0G 0B0
Canada

www.friesenpress.com

First Edition — 2022

ISBN
978-1-03-913546-8 (Hardcover)
978-1-03-913545-1 (Paperback)
978-1-03-913547-5 (eBook)

1. HEALTH & FITNESS, DISEASES, ALZHEIMER'S & DEMENTIA

Distributed to the trade by The Ingram Book Company

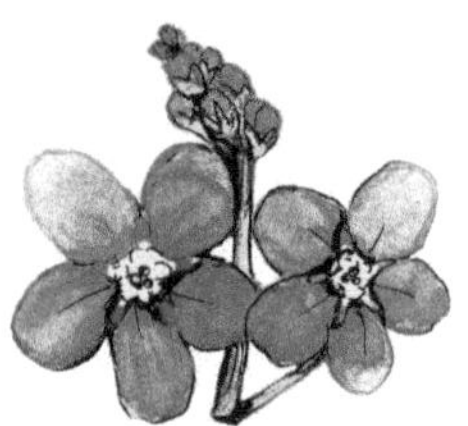

Acknowledgment

My dear Beth. I hope you can forgive me for divulging our innermost secrets of a very personal and distressing time in both our lives. I realize you were a very private person, and this book culminates into the biggest invasion of privacy anyone could ever propagate.

Know that I love you so much, and the only reason for this indiscretion is to perhaps help someone about to experience my pain and anguish, but more so, to perhaps help someone about to transgress into the confusion and frustration you had to endure.

In memory of the loving and caring person you were, if it helps but one person, I know you will approve; nonetheless, my shame for bringing your deviation from a normal life to light, cannot be excused. I felt; however, it had to be done. Please forgive me!

Everlasting words to Beth: The love we shared was extraordinary, and I so much want it to continue, alas, my wishes are all in vain. I know you are doing fine in a place with no pain, no confusion, no anxiety, and filled with all the love and happiness that rejoining with those preceding you can provide. Nonetheless, I am still here, suffering in your absence. I know for me it will end soon, and I will then rejoin you, but, until then… what do I do???

Till death do we reunite, my love!

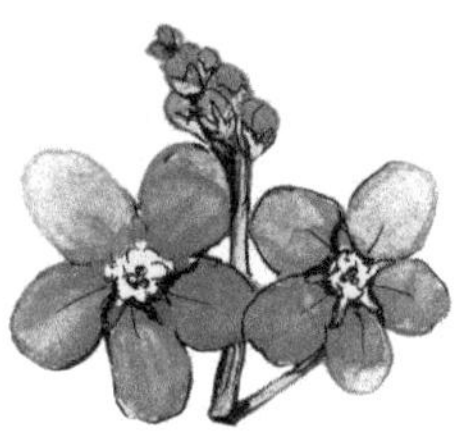

Prologue

THE NEED TO WRITE

Most people write because they know what they want to say! I felt I needed to write the accounts of one of the most tragic events to occur in my meager existence. The subject matter is very complex, comes with no instructions, and very little guidance. All I have is a layman's point of view with no expertise of what I'm writing about… I just know it's important.

The focus of this book is bewildering! Ever think of going on a vacation with no idea of where you're going, how long you will be away, not preparing, not packing, nor bringing anything with you? Then, while you're on this vacation, you don't know where you are, you're not sure how you got there, there is no path to follow, and the route ahead is pure fog. You have no idea of where you're headed and all you know is you need to take one step after another to just keep on going.

I do enjoy writing, nevertheless, I have no formal expertise on how to do so. I have a rather unique style; just don't expect to read enticing prose, eloquent grammar, or impeccable punctuation. I am an expressive talker with a lot of infliction in my voice, basically, I write like I talk. My writing style tends to have a flair for the dramatic, a penchant for the unusual, and a feeble attempt at comedy.

I'm not a journalist, that is my son's profession, so don't expect newsworthy facts and revelations on the subject matter. I'm a retired electronic technician with ten years in the Canadian Armed Forces, specifically the RCAF, followed by twenty-six years working for a telco. It seems ironic that currently, my son's hobby is repairing the mechanical and electronic workings of 1980s video games; conversely, I have taken to writing. He'll be the last one to assess this book as he would torture me with depressing memories of my failing Literature in Grade eleven.

I classify this book is a 'Pseudo–Sci-Spi Romantic Tragedy Memoir!!' Quite a mouthful! I reveal emotions and thoughts throughout my experiences on a subject matter that science knows something about and cannot yet change. It's not Sci-Fi because there is nothing fictitious about the subject matter. I say 'Spi' because I relied on my Spirituality, and how it carried me through this troubling time; perhaps, it is something that will assist you in your journey as well. For me this was a life changing event, and I simply want you to understand that my 'Spirituality' is referred to many times throughout this book as it has served me well.

My hope is to provide a degree of understanding for those about to experience this curse, to show you you're not alone, to provide insight into the psyche of what to expect, and to be thought provoking enough to help prepare you for the inevitable…all from the point of view of a loving male spouse.

I'm not a phycologist, I'm not a doctor, I'm not an author, although those professions would have helped! I don't have a university degree in anything, in fact, I didn't even graduate from high school.

So, what makes me qualified to write this book? I lost my soulmate to Alzheimer's!!

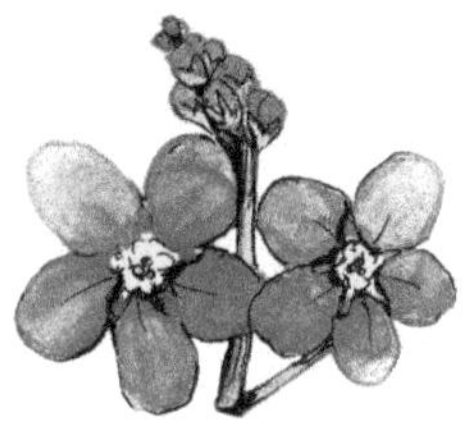

Precursor

I still love, and was once loved, by the most beautiful and precious soul on this earth. I am being biased of course… as are you, otherwise you would not be reading this book. When I show distress in a situation, I fully suspect that you will be feeling the same distress under the same conditions. For that reason, I am not going to dumb down my feelings to avoid any criticisms of being overly dramatic, highly emotional, displaying heightened anxieties, or even as being a wimp! Think of me as you will; however, if you relate to my emotions and accept that they are real and normal, then I have done my bidding; "Job well done, Art!!"

There are a few things you must understand about this book, it is not a book of instruction, nor a course on caregiving for an Alzheimer's patient. There are no questions at the end of every chapter, nor is there an exam at the end of the book. This is a recount of actual life experiences and reactions from a layman's point of view.

Case in point; it is currently two months before the third anniversary of Beth's passing, and I just discovered the term 'Aphasia'. It is a word that describes various types and stages of the inability of a patient to understand what is said and understood (receptive aphasia), then for them to be able to respond (expressive aphasia). The actual knowledge of aphasia would not have helped, and yet how to respond and manage aphasia would have helped immensely.

As you read on, you will clearly see that all I knew is that Beth became incoherent, and I was left high and dry. Some of my responses were curt, derogatory, and even placatory; it took time to learn, through experience, how to respond. I wish I would have known this aspect of Alzheimer's at the time; however, when you are consumed with the daily care, and the stress of anxiety regarding every aspect of your life and hers, there is little time to attend courses on caregiving. The fact that you are taking the time to read this book is a testament to the lack of preparation one has, and how desperate we are for knowledge.

The first thing I suggest you do is to join, and attend, Alzheimer's Support Group meetings, which generally run once a month in your region. If you can't find one, I suggest you start one. There are many people such as yourself in need. While attending the meetings the one thing that became very evident is that partners and caregivers of spouses with Alzheimer's were totally unprepared, and in bewilderment as to what was happening, what they needed to do, and how to do it.

A BIT ABOUT ME

Before I get into the issue at hand, namely Alzheimer's, I thought I should describe myself and my writing style as it will become quite evident that I am not a storyteller, all I can do is relate my experiences; I couldn't fabricate a story to save my life!

My writing style tends to be to document the occurrence with dialogues of depression, and/or delight, with somewhat of a theatrical flavour, combined with a flair for the dramatic. You'll find no William Shakespeare, Jules Vern, Mark Twain, or J.Y.Lilly here!! I guess you could call me the Van Gogh of authors.

You could consider me somewhat askew in the mental sense. I am fundamentally dyslexic; not in the 'Balk Tackwards, and get my Mords Wixed' sense, and I am just slightly dyslexic in the numerical sens (yeah, my dyslexic sister picked up the misspelling of the word 'sense', and thought the timing was hilarious).

'A genius is one that possesses a dyslexic mind with knowledge' (don't have a clue if this is true or not. It does; however, sound neat!!).

Obviously, I'm not a genius, and only partially dyslexic. Beth and I went to Mazatlán, Mexico with our son George for a vacation one year, and while there I needed a pair of sandals. Went to the local 'every shoe you've ever wanted' store and got a pair of Nike sandals. When I got back to the lodge, George said, "Nice Vikes!!" What can I say?? Besides, the 30 Pesos I overpaid was well worth it compared to the Shirkenbocks I was looking at.

I feel that finding Beth was a bit of Divine Intervention (no, I'm not trying to convert you, just my views on how, or why it happened). To begin with, on the day I was born, the Doctor…just kidding, not going back that far. I vividly remember thinking to myself that it was time to start looking for a wife back when I was in Grade three…for the second time. Grades one and two were schooled entirely in French, and when I changed town, and school, I was told that for Grade three, which was entirely in English, I would automatically fail. Heck, I could barely speak English much less write or read it.

After getting kicked out of school during Grade twelve for eating my lunch in the lunchroom (true story… why do these things happen to me?). I joined the Armed Forces and during my ten-year stint, I was able to connect with some wonderful women. I even proposed to three ladies, yet the thought of a transient lifestyle wasn't for them.

In March of 1976 I terminated my tenure in the Armed Forces, the second-best portion of my life, because of a dispute over the Francophone Status which I was trying to obtain. I was being passed over for promotion by French personnel with four years of service, they were now my superiors. I applied for Francophone Status, because of my ability to speak fluent French, and was rejected because "I didn't come from Quebec"!!! That was it!!! Screw them!! And again with 'Divine Providence', this time with direct and swift interaction.

AND NOW BETH (AND OUR SPECIAL FAMILY)

Upon getting released from the Armed Forces, and subsequently on my first day working as a Computer Technologist for Altel Data (an arm of AGT, now TELUS), I was tasked to do a 'ride-along' to learn the ropes. On that very first day I heard this beautiful enchanting voice of a dispatcher. Her demeanour was such that the techs on the radio were always trying to tease her, or at least taunt her to lose her cool, nevertheless, she would have none of it. In fact, rebuttal was always swift and with a pleasant mannerism, pushing right back at them. I thought to myself, "Now, there's a girl I would like to meet-up with! Ahh, but she's probably married… oh well!" (My exact thoughts).

About a year later, the Altel Data sales, dispatch, and technicians were merged as a group in a new building. The thought of this charming person never entered my mind, as I had grown so accustomed to her voice. One day, one of the clerks approached me and said, "someone in dispatch would like to go out with you". I was flattered and curious, and my comeback was, "Ok, who?" Regardless of my queries, she refused to divulge that information. My thought at the time was that a relationship with someone at work is never a good idea.

This matchmaking went on daily for a month or so, until I finally relented. She walked me up to Beth's desk and said, "Beth, Art would like to ask you something". Beth had no idea of what was happening, and you should have seen her blush when I asked her for a date, out loud, and in front of everyone else!!! My fate was sealed!!!

After dating Beth for a while, I was introduced to her son (George), and the most wonderful Grandma (Beth's) anyone could ever meet. It was a family situation I thoroughly enjoyed, and I, of course, proposed to Beth. After proposing, she related to me that George had nudged her and said, "Mom, don't let this one get away!" Thank you, Son!!!

An incident occurred while trying to organize our union that changed my views on religion. When I went to my Priest and told him I was going to marry Beth, whom had been divorced, I was told, "You cannot do that!" Reflecting on my past life, I felt that everything that had happened to me had led me to this juncture, and I wasn't about to miss out on this opportunity. I felt God wanted us together, and religious dogma was not going to prevent what was meant to be.

There was no doubt that this is what I wanted in life, dating back to Grade three when I decided it was time to find a wife. Beth, George, Nan (as she was known), and I were very close, and I knew I was making the right choice. My life with this wonderful family was so much better than I could have ever imagined! I cannot envision a more fulfilling, and rewarding life than that which I have experienced.

George was eight years old at the time, as I said, the product of a divorce. I knew I could never replace his dad, regardless of the situation that caused his parents to divorce. I also knew that George was the most important person in Beth's life; someone I could never replace. If he would have rejected me, the marriage would have never happened. It would have fulfilled my needs, and it would have fulfilled Beth's needs; nevertheless, it had to fulfill George's needs.

It is so important for people to know that!! You may love a woman, and she may love you; however, if there is any friction with a child, the marriage is probably doomed. If not, the psychological effect on the child will make both your lives unbearable and will probably result in unrepairable trauma to that child, to the point they self-destruct. That's why I insisted he become part of the wedding ceremony. It was crafted such that George walked Beth down the aisle, not to give away the bride, more so, for me to join the two of them as a family union. The preacher asked George if he accepted me into his family; likewise, if I accepted George as part of my family… we both said, "I Do!"

If he needed me to be a father figure, I would try to do that as best I could with my lack of experience! If he needed me to be a friend, I would do that! If I needed to mediate between mother and son, I was willing to do that, again, to the best of my capabilities, remaining neutral, with patience, empathy, and understanding. If he needed financial support, I would do that as well, and all these commitments extend to his wife, and of course, his kids. I was new to this fatherhood aspect in my life, fortunately for me George was very grounded, and there were no issues between us. We have a very strong family bond, something I wish all could experience. Though not related by bloodline, we are related in love!! See, love **is** thicker than blood!!

Once Beth was diagnosed with Alzheimer's, it occurred to me that divine intervention must have come into play, and I realized that this was my purpose in life. Everything that had ever happened to me prior to meeting Beth, the misguided youth, the unrequited love, the unfulfilled prayers, the death-defying stupidity, the career direction, and conversely, even her broken marriage had led to me marrying Beth; and now to care for her as she so deserved.

Some people feel that life is predestined, and every moment is preplanned in advanced. I don't believe that anything is preplanned. What would be the use of living without free will? What I believe is that, perhaps, the outcome is preplanned in that I feel Beth was my purpose in life, and Divine Providence guided, and protected me for this purpose. As I grew and learned, every nuance of caring I absorbed was a determining factor required to fulfill the task of caring for Beth, and as such, the guidance and protection that was afforded me to become Beth's caregiver; yes, even unrequited love…definitely the death-defying stupidity...I didn't mention my falling out of a third story window, did I? No tripping, no slipping, no pushing. In fact, there was no one else in the room. You might think 'off a deck' perhaps…but a window (I did mention stupidity, didn't I?)?? Anyways, perhaps fodder for another book, "Life Lessons Learned"?

But I digress, I never met George Sr., and never held anything against him. In fact, I felt so fortunate he gave Beth up for me that I thank the good Lord. I never discouraged George Jr. from seeking him out and reconnecting, the decision would be his. Unfortunately, it wasn't meant to be. George Sr. passed away about ten years after we were married. The main reason I mentioned George Sr. is to strengthen my case for divine providence.

Beth was loved by everyone; her smile was contagious and constant; a fun loving and adventurous lady with a great sense of humour, entwined with a great command of wit and wisdom. She had a perception of justice, and inclusion, that went above and beyond the norm. When someone (or I) would say, "Who cares??" she would respond with, "I care!!" If someone would criticize the rich, she would interject that, "It was a good thing some were rich, because they had the money to spend so as to keep people, and our economy, working!" She loved and would stand up for anyone, especially the 'under-dog'.

She was special, as all that knew her will attest!!! I believe that God knew this and cared deeply for this special angel. When she developed Alzheimer's, George Sr. would not have been around to care for her. Of course, our loving son would have gladly cared for her; however, he has a family of his own to support, and would not be able to devote all his time to her. I was the chosen one!! I feel very privileged that I was chosen by God, and that all the things that occurred in my life led me to become her support during this traumatic time for Beth. That's what I call divine Intervention, or providence, whichever you choose, and I feel so blessed!!

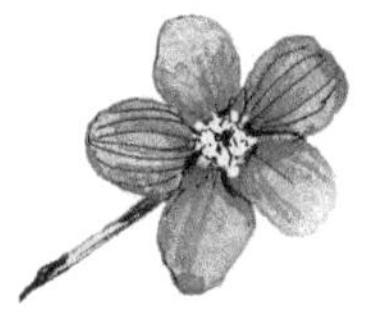

Chapter: The New Reality

This epic experience will take you on a journey like you have never been on and will likely change your life. You must be ready to forgo every aspect of your life and devote its entirety to the caregiving requirements you will now be faced with. Most men feel that beer, guns, and trucks are the essence of life. In this experience you will forget the big macho expression of the man you think you are, or want to be, and whittle yourself down to necessities of eating, sleeping, and caregiving with just dreams of entertainment, recreation, and reliving memories of days past. If you got what it takes, hang on, it's one hell of a ride; if you're self-absorbed, this book isn't for you… better turn tail and run, you're probably not man enough.

Each one of us is a different person with a different approach to life. If you are that big and burly macho man, this book may seem like hogwash. Nevertheless, if you truly love your spouse, loosen up and be prepared to experience the sorts of emotions that shake your soul! With true love of this unfortunate creature of yours, if in this book I don't make you tear up, your own experiences most likely will! Still with me? Deal with it, accept it, and get on with enjoying every diminishing, wonderful moment with your spouse while you still can.

Emotions are very personal, and you must realize that everyone will experience these emotions differently; each one of us feels love for their spouse differently; each one has different interactions with their spouse; and sadly, each one of us will experience different reactions emanating from your spouse within this disease.

The severity of these emotions is personal, and uniquely individual to each of us. They will vary from depression to elation for any incident. What causes those emotions, and how they evolve, are based on your knowledge of how events are transpiring, where things are going wrong, where things are going right, and how to handle any situations in particular. Perhaps I can provide you with a glimmer of hope, and an understanding of what you will be experiencing; perhaps even what action, or response to affect.

Unfortunately, I cannot provide any specific instructions, only observations and suggestions. With the stress, pain, and anxiety you feel, you will occasionally wonder if what you are doing is worth it; perhaps this book can answer that question.

The most important thing to remember is to react appropriately to these emotions! Any response of anger, or anxiety to an event, will impact the patient undesirably. You must have patience and accept that you must do what needs to be done without prejudice, judgment, ridicule, or objection… and this is from day one!!! If you must change, then change you must!

As my life began to dwindle, I felt it necessary to keep a journal of my experiences and mental state as I found it to be cathartic in an effort to keep my sanity. I found it necessary to write down what I was experiencing as if I was sharing with someone; in essence, I was sharing what was occurring and impacting me with myself as a venue of sorts. That led me to this autobiography of a life changing experience.

Emotions, as recorded, might seem dramatic and over inflated; nonetheless, with lack of previous experience at the time, were very real, and seemed very personal, poignant, and time sensitive; I make no apologies for being overly dramatic. Three years after Beth succumbing to Alzheimer's, that lack of previous experience still impacts my perception of life, and my emotional state has not diminished. I relive those emotions on a daily basis.

This is hell on earth, and although there is no actual hope, you must realize that you are not alone. Help, either supportive, or professional, is available where crying ***is*** expected and acceptable! Your sanity is worth far more than your ego.

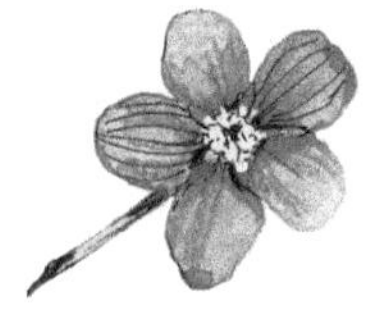

Chapter: Housekeeping

Alzheimer's has many facets and is very complex. What I present is but a narrow view of all the aspects of this disease. During my tenure as a caregiver for Beth, there were many observations I made where, had I known of and expected these peculiarities, my reaction to, and the outcome of my experiences, could have been vastly different. As such, the purpose of this book is to try to elaborate on all the thoughts that proliferated my mind before, during, and after what I lived through with the loss of my soulmate; I reflect on all those thoughts to help prepare you for what might be coming in your journey.

There are a few items we need to get out of the way, specifically for your benefit. First and foremost, the most important thing you must do is to get your affairs in order… ASAP! I can't stress enough how important Estate Planning to be. In addition to Estate Planning, with the diagnosis and imminent onset of Alzheimer's, there are housekeeping issues such as finances, the potential impact of a mishaps, and planning for placement in a care facility to be aware of and be prepared for.

For those beginning this journey, it is very important that you now review these housekeeping issues (actually, these so called 'housekeeping issues' pertain to diagnosis of any debilitating disease, not just Alzheimer's). I encourage you to now divert your attention to the back of this book, to the Addendum labelled 'Housekeeping' before you proceed with this romantic tragedy I am about to unfold.

Upon your return from said 'Addendum', although the following observations and comments are not actually housekeeping aspects, you might be about to, and/or already have, experienced some of the following peculiarities. These reflections, though relevant to Alzheimer's, are not necessarily linked to my situation with Beth; nonetheless, I felt it best to review the following remarks before we get into the crux of the matter; that being the experiences of my specific situation. Please read on!!

TRANSITIONING

Every Alzheimer's patient will experience changes differently in the transition from the person you knew, to the person she is becoming; it's not an exact science. My experiences are the only thing I can recount with any validity, and in my case, taking care of Beth was all inclusive, peaceful, and very acceptable to deal with. It was my choice to devote my priorities to her care; as such, found the process to be fraught with ever deepening emotions and anxiety, culminating in an unrelenting state of love and devotion on my behalf.

Had I known what she was about to experience, I could have been prepared for Beth's regression, and I would have known what to expect, and known how to respond, both physically and verbally. I could have had less anxiety and be able to sit back and let things occur AS WAS EXPECTED! I could have enjoyed every, last, precious moment with my Beth and coddled her into regression as if growing old together…as I so wanted to do! Alas, now I live in remorse with the memories, questioning if I could have done something to ease her confusion, her anguish, and ease my anxiety, my guilt… had I known.

There are other forms of transformation to be considered. When I mention to others of Beth's passing on, due to Alzheimer's, I find it disturbing that many people relate, as a first comment, the account of violence and anxiety projected by patients. This seems to be a prevalent situation. Patients that are the most loving and caring people you could ever want to meet, turn into someone you have never wanted to know.

With this psychological perspective as a consideration, a loving person could transition into an abusive partner and culminate into the requirement to have local authority step in, perhaps transpiring into your loved one being committed to a hospital, or a continuing care facility. Of course, this would be more predominant, though not exclusive to a male patient, a consideration, nonetheless.

So, why would a person transform into the total opposite of their previous being? There are many reasons! If aggression is prevalent in your loved one, I suggest you get professional help regarding this situation as soon as you can.

I attended a virtual seminar provided by the AsantCafé as part of the Alzheimer's Society in Alberta, Canada, labeled "Feeling's of Needs and Expression's" [1]. Excerpts from this presentation are reflected, with creative license, as follows.

You must not forget that changes have occurred in their brain, and these will affect every persona of the person you once knew regarding memory, mood, and behavior amongst other attributes. First thing I would suggest is to assess if there has been a sudden change in environment or medication, or has the onset been gradual?

Changes you are observing may be a form of expression that you are unfamiliar with, and yet, perhaps the only way a patient can communicate as they lose their ability to formulate relevant sentences and/or even be able to speak at all. Imagine the frustration of not being understood when you are hungry, or you have a need to go to the bathroom and not be able to find the facilities. Just these two simple requirements in life could result in anxiety, wandering, or even the aggression we speak of.

In most cases, the patients are responding to some sort of stimuli, regardless of how simple it might have been. It could be in response to the body language you use, maybe the way you speak to them, or what you say, perhaps

1 Feeling's of Needs and Expression's presentation by Jeannine Chemello RPN

new medications, or even their perception of a new caregiver. For a person that has always been a private person to suddenly be given a bath by a stranger might be unimaginable; now imagine if that person is of the opposite gender.

Another consideration is that there are countless instances of repressed feelings that phycologists attribute to abuse or neglect as a child. A patient might be regressing into the memory of their childhood during their teenage years, or from a male perspective, as a football star, perhaps as a hunter, or worse, a Kung Fu student. When the patient regresses, and are living in the past, perhaps they were being bullied, or perhaps were a bully, and that is now first and foremost in their mind. They may be reacting to those memories as the current reality. This consideration relates to their past, which hopefully you will be aware of, and be able to use as a clue pertaining to what, or why, these changes are occurring.

You must also consider that perhaps, there have always been latent tendencies of jealousy, intimidation, or insecurity in your relationship. In the normal situation that we call life, those tendencies might have been suppressed for the good of all, or even as a sign of wellbeing. This is where you must look within! Perhaps she wanted a life of living in the arts, or even knitting, whereas you provided a life of fishing and hunting, that she accepted and repressed out of love for you. You might have displayed negative tendencies throughout your union that she has supressed until now. I'm not trying to say you were at fault, more so as a reason for her transition; it is a possibility to consider. Once supressed tendencies become the new reality of a confused mind, they come to the forefront, and all hell breaks loose. Regardless, physical aggression must be understood and managed; appropriate action must be taken.

Other reasons that might propagate transitions, relate to the unfamiliarity of being moved to a new location. Being removed from your home, and not understanding why, is very traumatic for anyone. With this consideration in mind, can you imagine a situation where the loved ones in the patient's life are unable to stay with, or even visit the patient for days or weeks on end? Absence could be through no fault of your own due to work requirements, or other family situation, or unfortunately, for your own specific reasonings and/or desires. "I can't handle this impingement on my life!!! See you later sweetie!!" In a confused mind, this will become a definitive sign of abandonment. Don't expect the patient to understand ANY reasoning, valid or not.

Reflecting on my own experience, I can only feel compassion for these patients in that they might not be ushered through their disease with the love and compassion they deserve as the beautiful and loving persons they once were.

You perhaps have, or will have, a lot of anxiety of your own if, and/or when, these disturbing patterns evolve. The care you would want to provide could become unbearable. My only hope is that you can find some sort of methodology in care that helps resolve, or at least ease, your personal situation.

What concerns me most, and the reason I want to address psychological transformations towards the beginning of this book, is that if this is what you are experiencing, this book will not necessarily address nor help you in this situation. There is a lot of support you can get on this subject from The Alzheimer's Society, or if in distress, call 811

(Caveat: available in Canada; not aware what is available in the rest of the world).

DENIAL

Lastly, one of the side effects of a physical, or psychological transition, potentially one of the worst things to happen to you and your spouse, is 'Denial'. Unfortunately, this happens very often, and it can come from many sources; you, your spouse, relatives, and even the medical profession; all can propagate some forms of denial. This is something that, at this juncture, I must devote some referencing comments.

In the onset, you will question whether your loved one 'actually has' dementia, and would like definitive assurance of the diagnosis. Unfortunately, denial due to this doubt, will persist even after diagnosis in that positive diagnosis will not come from the medical profession! It's common knowledge, and I feel one of the worst things to hear from the medical profession, is that "the only way to diagnose dementia is through autopsy after death". That's what I was told! It's not hard enough to grasp the reality of the situation, that they now throw in a degree of uncertainty and anguish for the rest of your spouse's life. The last thing I wanted to hear, once she had passed away, was "Yep, she had Alzheimer's!" as if I didn't know. Worse yet would be, "Oops, we were wrong! It was a kidney infection." Can you imagine the guilt??

A more prevalent form of denial will emanate from your spouse. More than likely, your spouse will be in denial because she cannot sense the difference in her own behavior. At times she will even blame you for the confusion she will experience. It is imperative to not take this personally! It will be a hurtle that is very hard to overcome, and adjust to… and it is you that must adjust.

Another instance of denial you might encounter could come from relatives. This has the potential of disrupting, or even destroying, your relationship with them, or worse, with your spouse. The knowledge of Alzheimer's being potentially hereditary and perceived as an affront on the 'all important family name', can be relevant, prevalent, and thereby denounced. Thankfully most won't, nonetheless, this could result in blaming you for fabricating this disease upon their relative. Suggesting placement in a care facility would be 'absurd' to them.

SELF-DENIAL

The worst, and most destructive form of denial, is your own denial in that your spouse has been inflicted with this disease. Within this form of denial, there are different ways you will handle this affront on your life, and none of them are good.

You might use 'avoidance' in that 'if you don't deal with it, it will go away'. This occurrence of denial is altogether too customary, and very destructive to the patient. This form of denial will, of course, be more prevalent at the beginning stages of dementia due to the lack of knowledge regarding the disease, and what it is doing to the one you have loved, known, and respected for the last thirty years or so.

Unfortunately, one appalling form of your denial is 'blame', in that you notice the changes and start blaming her for every unusual thing she does as being 'different and unacceptable'! This is what most would categorize as abuse! She will feel that it is her fault you are rejecting her, an agony I can only imagine as you criticize her every little mistake. "What the heck is the matter with you?"; "Can't you even cook supper, or clean the house??"; "Where's my beer??" … tragic!! It's not the way to treat the one you love!

Worst case scenario, as a result of self-denial, would be 'Abandonment', and is one consideration of denial you might consider. You will question if it would be better for you if you just walked away, and of course it would be… if you are only concerned for yourself. The reason you were united in the first place was for the mutual benefit provided to both of you. To abandon your spouse now, is a reflection of your being self-involved, to the point of considering only the things that matter to you. Think of how she feels when she depended, relied, and felt secure in your presence, and suddenly, she cannot understand why you are not there when she needs you most; adding to the confusion she is experiencing.

The thing you may not be considering, is the guilt you will be subject to if you do decide to leave! I reflected on such thoughts, my life was in shambles and not getting any better; regardless, I would never have abandoned Beth. It would have relieved me of a lot of stress and bewilderment; nevertheless, I held on to the end willingly. I know I did the right thing; I know I did the best I could, and yet, I am still haunted by some form of neglect of onus. I ***can not***, for one moment, imagine the guilt I would feel if I had abandoned Beth, something I would not be able to live with; that, my friend, is a serious consideration for yourself.

Hopefully, for your spouse's sake, I can help you decide to stay, and I am able to make that decision bearable. This disease may be devastating for you, nonetheless, how do you think it is for your spouse? What she needs most is love, understanding, security, and patience, not accusations, avoidance, abandonment, nor any other form of denial.

There will be good times if you look for them. Beth and I had many smiles, laughs, and lots of tender moments five years after diagnosis. Don't grieve the one you love before you've lost them; treasure every moment together while you can.

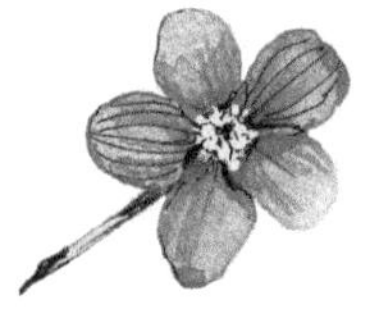

Chapter: Preliminary Observations

For me this story started ten years ago, slowly, subtly, and with no advanced warning. I suspected nothing, was happy with my lot in life, and could not want for more. Little did I know it was all about to change, and how little nothing else but Beth's happiness, care, and security mattered. Here goes!!

I noticed subtle differences in her capabilities for almost two years before I started the journal of events; many of the changes I attributed to aging, some to just plain being weird. Watching my true love disintegrate before my eyes had a great impact on my emotional state. There were many doubts as to what I was observing, what was going on, what was going to happen next, yet mostly what I was expected, or needed to do. Most disturbing was the lack of information on the assessment of these changes.

In the beginning Beth didn't act in the stereotypical manner you see in movies, wherein the person starts to misplace things, are confused regarding where they are, forgetting where they put things like their keys, wandering off someplace and getting lost, cooking and leaving burners on, or forgetting people close to them. Purportedly symptoms of forgetfulness, absentmindedness, wandering, repetition, and confusion depicted in the Hollywood movies as being the first signs of dementia. Maybe Hollywood brings them into the forefront to establish cases of dementia as a storyline.

In movies you'll notice that in most cases it is a person that visits occasionally that sees these peculiarities. Perhaps I didn't notice these subtle changes because we were inseparable, always doing things together. We were not the 'I'm going Golfing while you stay home and Knit' types; not to say that there is anything wrong with that whatsoever. We had similar desires, and that is what made Beth and I so close as a couple. Knowing where your comfortable level is with each other is the essence of being soulmates.

In Beth's case the above-mentioned symptoms never seemed to appear as much as I thought would be the norm. Some of these symptoms materialized much later in the process, and by then I understood what might be taking place. Beth's symptoms were more out of the blue where suddenly she would do something very strange and then be normal for days on end.

The first occurrence I can recall of uncharacteristic behaviour, is when I was in the kitchen, at three in the morning, and Beth came out of the bedroom, went to the garbage can, which sat at the end of the island, lifted the lid and began to squat. My mind raced at realization of this situation, and I thought perhaps she was sleepwalking, even though her eyes were open.

As I'm sure you are aware, they say you should never awaken someone that is sleepwalking. Though this ran through my mind, this was a dire situation that needed immediate attention. I think I said something like, "No, no, Honey, not there... come with me to the washroom"; I then guided her in the proper direction. What seemed unusual was that it didn't seem to awaken her, and she remained in a trance of sorts. The peculiarity was averted, all was well as she went back to bed without saying a word.

What really started my concern over the unusual, was my lack of comprehension whereby I just couldn't understand where she was coming from. I would occasionally notice Beth would become emotionally overly sensitive or become mentally detached in that she would become reserved, and in a seemingly different world. Subsequently, I would react in a normal, corrective, defensive manner, or I would question why she was avoiding my presence; everything had to be according to normality after all.

We never did argue much, and early on it seemed out of character that I'd get accused of being mad, or shouting, seemingly out of the blue. I've always been an expressive talker, and change in the inflection or expression in my voice would bring on these accusations. That's when many times an argument would ensue while trying to defend myself or profess my innocence. The realization of what was going on took quite a while, until I figured out that there was something wrong, and I didn't always have to be correct nor be so anal.

That was the first change I started making; let her win because it just wasn't worth the argument, or the victory. The words "yes dear" we're used a lot, and I now realize how demeaning that must have been until it actually started working to reduce conflict. I started using those words with affection and understanding in that it caused less anxiety for both of us. This was about the time the possibility of dementia came into focus.

She was always open and friendly, even with strangers. She had a killer smile that calmed your soul and warmed your heart. She was outgoing, and would talk freely to anyone; that's where her social skills and sense of humor would shine. Eventually I noticed her demeanour changing from being confident and self-assured to being self-conscious and timid. She started to become reserved and withdrawing from society, and not wanting to go places nor do things. She would shy away from having any attention focused her direction, even with extended family and friends, and especially when in public.

Ultimately, this was the main, in fact, the only reason we had to remove ourselves from the Lion's Club. The Lion's Club depends entirely on the involvement and participation of its members. It broke my heart when we had to resign, loosing social contact with the friends we had acquired. I believe she was withdrawing from society as well as acquaintances because she was a very proud and private lady. The thought of someone having pity for her was inconceivable.

At some point, I noticed that she would always walk behind me. I'm not sure why, and I tried to encourage her to walk arm and arm with me. In a crowded area she would always drop back and follow. Normally people are protective of their personal space when they feel they have a right to be there;

however, she became reserved, and didn't want to get in anyone's way! She would even apologize to people in a lineup behind us, for cutting in front of them when we were clearly first in line.

One thing's for sure, there were a lot more hugs and kisses. I took every opportunity that presented itself to enjoy her affection while I could, and I felt she responded well to our little moments. It felt great to hold her hand or go arm in arm in public, even getting in a peck or two, and it made her smile. We did a lot of this at home as well, and it felt great. Even passing in the hallway rarely went by without a smooch.

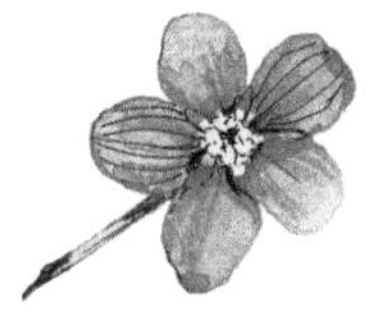

Chapter: The Timeline

This book is arranged as a timeline of events that has restructured my life into a new reality. I can't tell you how to fix or counteract what is happening to your spouse; there is nothing that can be done to avert that course of development. Best I can do is prepare you for what might happen.

Most of the dates are chronological as documented. I will; however, be going back in memory to the perception of how and when the changes were occurring. At times, I had to interject a few current memories as they seemed pertinent and time sensitive for continuity.

The following observations reflect my then current demeanour, as it was happening, and may at times seem lengthy and repetitive. I felt it pertinent to leave those comments in as a recurrence of that effect, and to strengthen its relevancy. My main hope is that you don't get bored with the redundancy. If I reiterate a hundred times that she got upset because I turned left, it's because it's directly proportional to the frequency of the occurrence, proportional to the time span between occurrences, and that's how many times you can expect the same reaction; it reflects how superfluous your life might become. Just be thankful I didn't repeat it in a simple point format:

- A week ago, she got mad at me!
- Yesterday, she got mad at me!
- Today, she got mad at me again!
- Tomorrow…you guessed it!!

Come to think of it, that's sort of what I will be doing…sorry!

Perhaps you can gain insight into some of the situations you are currently facing or will be experiencing, and you can somehow avoid falling into some of the pitfalls as I did. I am trying to project what to expect or perhaps what is to come…something I was not privileged to.

The situations revealed in the preceding chapter, were preliminary and gradual in the onset of Alzheimer's, and occurred over the period of a year… approximately. At the time, I was unsure what was taking place and/or the reasoning behind the incidences; following is more specific to the time and occurrence to which I can attach a date.

21 JULY, 2012

Strange occurrences of forgetfulness and uncharacteristic behaviour were starting to emerge well before this date, and this is pretty much the time I felt the need to start this journal.

We were invited to friends for dinner. During the afternoon, Beth seemed a little distant. She was wandering around the yard, and didn't hang around with me, as she normally would have, while we socialized and had a beer around the firepit.

It was supper time, or dinner if you choose, and fortunately, I was sitting kitty corner from Beth at the table. While we were serving the food dishes, she suddenly put her hand in the potato salad serving dish, and food went straight to her mouth. I intervened, and dished out the proportions for her. This was quite a shock to our friends, as they had no idea what was going on… at the time, neither did I. We did; however, take the incident in stride. I seemed to instinctively know that if I acted up in anyway, there could be lots of issues.

I then realized her using utensils was troublesome. She could not she use the knife to cut her food, so I proceeded to cut the food for her, allowing her to use her fork. I knew something was up prior to this event, I had noticed changes that were not simply 'minor occurrences' that could be considered as just 'getting old'. My worst fears were now confirmed.

It then became very evident that she seemingly couldn't formulate a coherent sentence. The sudden incapability to convers horrified me, and all I could think of was that this was it; the best I could expect going forward. Boy was I wrong! Alzheimer's isn't quite so linear, and the path not so foreseeable.

Needless to say, the evening didn't last long. Once supper was over, I felt the need to excuse ourselves. I would discuss what occurred with our friends later.

2 AUG, 2012

Went to our local GP to assess what was happening. You can't imagine the distress when you realize something is not right with your partner, and you need to get it analyzed by a medical practitioner, and yet, how can you involve the person you love, and divulge your intent? It is best for your spouse, nevertheless, feels like you are throwing her under the bus… as they say.

This is the first time these issues regarding dementia were to be addressed. Problem being, Beth and I always go in the doctor's office together, and that doesn't allow me to come right out and discuss the situation with the doctor. I can't directly ask the doctors to assess Beth for Alzheimer's without having Beth retaliate. In order to circumvent any anxiety, I suggested to Beth that we both undergo an assessment of our health under the guise of a yearly checkup. I had realized that Beth was not acting 'normally' for a while now; in reality, I wanted to identify any potential problems with her, and with myself as well. The exam showed that there were inconsistencies regarding Beth's comprehension and memoir, yet nothing could be verified at the time. Beth was scheduled for another appointment for a 'Mental Assessment' (what a terrible and terrifying terminology).

It is a devastating diagnosis to hear, and now is not the time to be in denial. It's the beginning of a new world for you and your spouse, and it is better to know what the reality is. It is also time to seek out the resources you need to deal with the issues as they arise… and that they will!!

As an addendum: Why did it feel at the time that I was condemning Beth to this terrible disease? Why didn't I wait till things get out of hand? Was it that I wanted this to happen to her? Of course, the answer to the last question is 'NO!'; nevertheless, these thoughts went through my mind.

6 AUG, 2012

Assessment time. It went well, and the Nurse was very accommodating to Beth regarding the test purpose and results. Yep, something is up! Assessment review with the GP did not go as well. There are result numbers that meant nothing to me, and I don't recall what they were; in retrospect, I wish I had recorded them. The GP identified a potential issue, and rescheduled a follow-up for another assessment for Beth.

14 AUG, 2012

Leaving her alone:

It's gotten to the point where I don't dare leave her alone while shopping, or even ask her to meet me somewhere. I can still leave her in an area, and tell her I'll be back. Coordinating a meeting spot; however, is out of the question.

The scariest moment to occur, was when she went to the washroom while we were in the UofA Hospital visiting my mom. We were just down the hall, and unfortunately, I didn't notice her emerging from the washroom. She went the wrong direction, and got lost for over an hour. I searched frantically for her; nonetheless, was nowhere to be found. Imagine if you will, loosing someone in a place where she looks like she belongs, and she's unable to tell you where she came from, who she is, nor even whom she's visiting. There are many floors, hallways, corridors, rooms, not to mention the doors leading outside. I was frantic!!! Had to call security to have her description given over the PA system. Security eventually found her, and brought her back. She was not going to get out of my sight ever again!

11 SEPT, 2012

The next assessment confirmed there was an issue, potentially Alzheimer's. We had Beth leave the room so the Doc and I could discuss things in private. Worst part of the consultation was that this GP is loud, and Beth could hear everything that was being discussed.

My world was unravelling before my eyes!!! I asked, "What could be done?", or at least "What's next?" He said there were medications available to help stabilize the onset, although, these would not cure or even postpone the inevitable. "When?"…5 to 20 years!!

Beth was very reserved on the way home. I'm not sure she understood what the prognosis was. I was terrified as to what I would say or have to say!!! Can't recall what happened, my mind was in a haze, we were good nonetheless.

An appointment was set up with a neurologist. Till then, there were ongoing assessments with the same results, and still a lack of helpful information.

I find the hardest thing to deal with right now is explaining to people what's happening. Beth is very smart, and I believe she knows what is happening. She is also sensitive, and gets really upset if she thinks I, or someone, is talking behind her back. Even to this day she's very selective as to whom should know about her Cancer, a year after it's been beaten.

Many people have noticed her changes, and I don't know what to say behind her back, ironic as it may sound. It seems funny, the people closest to her don't seem to notice the changes. Until there is a clear diagnosis, I don't want to suggest an issue (again, reminiscent of talking behind her back).

As it turned out Beth didn't want anyone to know she had Alzheimer's; in fact, she forbade me to tell anyone after her diagnosis. She dreaded the look of pity and sorrow in her friends and relatives' eyes, and didn't want to be treated any differently than before. That, in of itself, was one of the hardest things to deal with. I know this was a personal preference and not denial; although, she did go into denial as time went on. At one point she argued that the neurologist specifically told her she **didn't** have Alzheimer's. I found it would be very hard to tell her, or insist, she had Alzheimer's, so I didn't; in fact, I avoided ever speaking that word again in her presence.

23 SEPT, 2012

My mom passed away today; she was sixteen days shy of her ninetieth birthday. Such a sweet, wonderful woman, and yet, underappreciated on my behalf, for which, I am so sorry!

Dad was wheelchair bound at the time, and during the funeral I had to maneuver him into the facilities to help him, which took the better part of an hour. As such, I had to leave Beth alone, and in the care of my siblings; all went well. Beth seemed to understand, and there were no issues to speak of during the funeral. Beth loved my mom, and I could tell she felt a sense of loss as well.

OCT 28TH, 2012

It's starting to get serious now. I had to go to Panorama for a Board Meeting and Beth was going to stay with her mom in Calgary from Monday till Wednesday. I was concerned, nonetheless figured she would be OK.

Before we left home, I reviewed how to use the cellphone, and how to find my number using the contacts list. Beth couldn't grasp the concept, and decided to write the numbers down. She couldn't remember my number, which didn't surprise me too much. What did surprise me is when she couldn't remember her mom's number, a number that she dials almost every other day.

I was extremely relieved when, once we left home, she decided to come with me. I know I said I would never let her get out of my sight, yet I figured she'd be OK with her mom; it is now to the point where I will not leave her alone with anyone, even for a day.

NOV 18, 2012

Just to show we do have good days, we watched the CFL semi-finals today. Beth was quite OK with that. After the game, I suggested we watch a Kung Fu movie… Beth said "Yeah, I'd like to see that girl in 'Scratching Cow, Biting Pig'!"… her actual words, LOL.

At times, completing sentences are becoming harder and harder for her to formulate, and she has become aware of this. Finishing her sentences for her, as we all tend to do with familiarity, confuses her, and breaks her train of thought. Trying to suggest what she is trying to say doesn't work very well either, keep that in mind. When I question what she was trying to say, it either results in an aggressive answer, or she will say she was "just joking, can't you take a joke?" I now realize that she must feel embarrassed, as such, that is a defensive response on her behalf.

This is where I now must try to let her formulate her own sentences, agree with her (yes dear), or choose my words very well, empathize, and acknowledge that I understand how difficult it must be for her to communicate ("That's OK dear, don't worry about it") ("Yeah, it's confusing for me too"). The hardest part now is watching my every word, every infliction in my voice, and how I question her reasoning in an effort to understand her.

NOV 22, 2012

What a day!!!

I knew it was going to be an interesting day from the start. We had to visit dad, and I could tell that Beth was having a 'confusion day'.

Beth had wandering sentences all day; she intertwined multiple thoughts into one sentence continually. I can't remember the actual words, nonetheless, the situation is scary; how can I respond? I try for clarity, yet she can't straighten things out, and goes into "I'm joking", or "oh never mind" mode. I'm sure the latter is because she realizes she isn't able to say what she intends to say.

She had difficulty scheduling time and events. We made a haircut appointment for dad at his continuing care centre for 1:15 p.m. as we were leaving to go for lunch at 11:30 a.m. We started loading dad into the van and Beth, turned dad's wheelchair around to go for the haircut. I tried to explain that we had an hour and forty-five minutes before dad was getting the haircut, and we were going for lunch first, nonetheless, she insisted we had to go for the haircut immediately. It took quite a while to convince her otherwise; she was visibly upset as we were leaving.

At one time, while unloading dad, she tried to buckle the front passenger seat belt into the rear seat buckle.

For the first time, I noticed she was hearing things today, all day long. At one time while heading home, she tried to turn the volume up on the radio to listen to something; however, the radio was off. She even tried to tell me what she thought she heard; unfortunately, it didn't make any sense. Out of the blue, she then said something like "So that's it then? It doesn't matter what they're saying?" (Not exact words). She was implying that I turned the radio off, even though it hadn't been on for about twenty minutes… I turned it on.

As it was extremely hard to handle both Beth and dad today, I wish I could have record today's events, as they happened; however, it wasn't possible. I went into a state of depression for most of the day; even dad noticed. We were having a coffee when back at the continuing care centre, and while Beth had gone to the washroom, dad looked at me and said, "What are you thinking?" He could tell something was wrong; I could see it in his eyes. I hesitated for a while; tears started to well-up in my eyes. I just about told him what was going on; all I could think of was to change the subject. I said, "Oh, just thinking of Mom", an already touching subject.

I'm having a hard time coping with all this. At times I want to go into seclusion and get drunk! I know it's a fleeting thought, and won't resolve anything. I feel I can't handle this! I want to be left alone, free of this burden, yet realize I can't.

7 DEC, 2012

My unhappy birthday! By now it has become obvious to friends and relatives that something is afoot with Beth. I have been asked many times, and I can no longer deny any issues. This wasn't a large gathering; nevertheless, when we could separate from Beth, and of course behind Beth's back, I disclosed the situation. I think there was some relief, yet, mostly acceptance by some; regardless, it is a hard pill to swallow. There had been some suspicion by most, and once the truth was revealed the mood at the gathering changed noticeably. They asked, "What can be done?" "What can we do?" The obvious answers are "Nothing!", and "Don't treat Beth any differently".

I couldn't leave people in the dark any longer, revealing Beth's diagnosis was the 'de facto' answer I was to provide going forward. It wasn't like I was broadcasting to the world; however, I felt there was no need to continue the charade, and allay their thoughts that I must be in denial. The reveal went quite well, compared to what could have occurred. Their cognisance of the situation was found to be helpful in dealing with Beth on all our behaves.

Once relatives realize that Alzheimer's is the obvious diagnosis, fear amongst family members comes into play, and some will turn to you as the foremost expert for reassurance that they, themselves, will be spared. This does add greatly to the stress, something that you don't need. It's hard to tell someone that you "just don't know", and much easier to reassure them not to worry in the hopes that they will be spared the Alzheimer's bullet.

I find it ironic that if you reassure them, and ease their anxiety, they will ultimately be the last to know they have Alzheimer's because of the ways Alzheimer's progresses. Upon reading this, my relatives will probably be cursing me for what I've just written; nonetheless, I relate a relevant story regarding being diagnosed with Alzheimer's towards the end of this book; check out the fourth paragraph in the Chapter called 'Finding Solace'… you might want to jump ahead and review it before sending me hate mail.

16 DEC, 2012

Beth is losing all concept of timing. Today we were invited to our son's place for Christmas, tonight she started to pack to get ready to go at 11:00 p.m.; we're not expected until the 24th. It was difficult to explain to her that we weren't expected for a couple days so I suggested we finish packing in the morning. By then it wasn't an issue.

17 DEC, 2012

The most surprising thing to occur to date was this morning at about 6:30 a.m., Beth got out of bed and put her new glasses in the microwave, instead of her magic bag. For at least half an hour afterwards, she couldn't understand why the magic bag had somewhat melted thinking the glasses were the magic bag, even with the burnt glasses in front of her. She even thought I helped her turn the microwave on. This is bad!! I can't keep her away from the microwave in the middle of the night, so I'll have to keep it unplugged. There is still an issue with the stove; however, she doesn't use it alone as we do most of the cooking together; she rarely uses the stove to just heat something up.

DEC 18, 2012

Well, it's been a bad 3 days, and things are getting worse. Beth has lost all concept of timing with respect to dates of events, and when we need to prepare for those commitments. She is aware of what needs to be done, yet oblivious as to when we need to proceed, or even start preparing for the event.

I've been busy committing to being Santa Claus for the local community, and I can't do that anymore. Beth is integral in the appearance, and was dressed at 5:30 a.m. for a gig in the afternoon, a good six hours before we are supposed to be there. It was difficult explaining that we weren't ready to leave, and even that we had to eat first.

The thing that occurs to me is that she consistently will remember scheduled events with no concept of timing. It might put off a lot of frustration if I simply do not divulge events prior to the time to prepare…just a thought in retrospect.

THE SANTA CLAUSE [2]

To steel the title from Tim Allen's Movie, and yet to capture its significance, taking on Alzheimer's seemed akin to the focus of said movie. The concept being that being Santa Claus was forced upon Tim Allen, under a clause in a contract that he must replace the Santa he just irradicated; isn't much different than suddenly being told that the woman you love, and are so compatible with, will now be transformed into a completely different person that you will not recognize. More so, you are now put to task, within this

2 ***The Santa Clause*** is a 1994 American Christmas comedy film written by Leo Benvenuti and Steve Rudnick, and directed by John Pasquin.

commitment, to completely change your own perspective on your life from the one you were totally in tune with to one of total caregiving dedication.

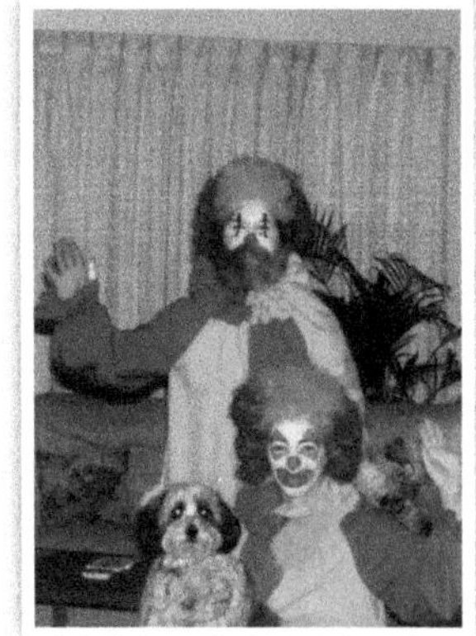

What started my foray into the world of the Santa, was a Halloween candy giving experience that blew my mind. I was standing at our front door, handing out candies, dressed as a clown with a multi-coloured curly plastic wig on my head, a painted clown face with green and yellow died (painted) natural beard, and supporting a clown costume. While a mother, and a 4-year-old child, were at the door, the child's eyes were fixated on me, and she never said a word. I thought she might have been frightened with the fear that so many people have of clowns that so persists into adulthood. Pleasant as I tried to be, she never flinched a smile. Upon leaving, with the child constantly staring at me, looking back in a locked fixation, at about 20 feet away she turned to her mother and asked, "Mom, was that Santa Claus?" I was blown away!!! After that time, I just couldn't let it rest, and played on the recognisance throughout the year for years to come.

I was the perfect Santa Claus. A five-foot four-inch Elf with a paunch and gold rimmed glasses. I also had the canny ability to converse with children of all ages, even teenagers, and was never stumped for an answer on a question they had posed so as to validify my authenticity. Most striking was that I also supported a beard that was the envy of most shopping mall Santa's, even those with real beards. Turns out, though my hair is still brownish, with hillites of grey as the distinguished older gentleman I am, my beard is fluffy and perfectly white. When adults ask, "what gives?", I would reply, "I have no idea… my beard is eighteen years younger than my hair!!"

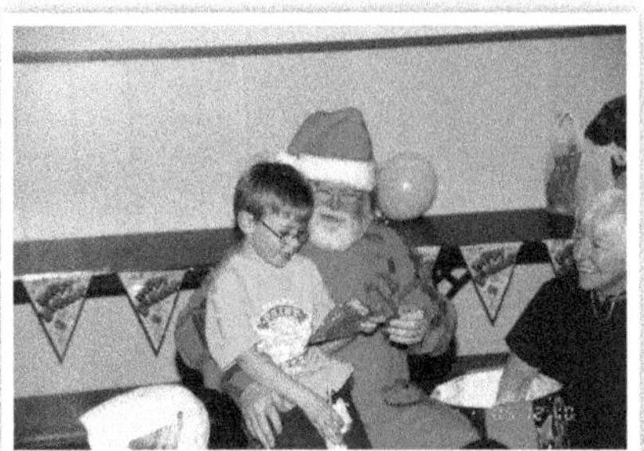

During a July vacation, at the Johnson Canyon Hot Springs, situated on the Trans-Canada highway in BC, while in the swimming pool, wearing a bathing suit (not even red), I caught a glance of a six years old boy, staring at me in wonder. I waved him over, to which his parents approved, and asked him, "Do you know who I am?" He nodded a distinct "No!", so I told him I was Santa Claus. A smile of acknowledgement painted itself across his face, then a look of bewilderment to which I added, "I'm on vacation!" Well, I soon became the hit of the swimming pool, with all the kids surrounding me and asking questions regarding everything from whether Beth was Mrs. Santa Claus, to where the reindeers were. It was fantastic!!

It was a natural progression that I became the Rimbey Santa, and Beth became Mrs. Claus for five years, entertaining kids at Santa parades, kindergarten classes, store engagements, Christmas celebrations at community halls, and many private events. I even appeared at a hatrurite colony; I was a hit with the kids…not so much with the elders. I fully respect their beliefs, and didn't mean to overstep my bounds; however, it was done through an invitation with no ill intent.

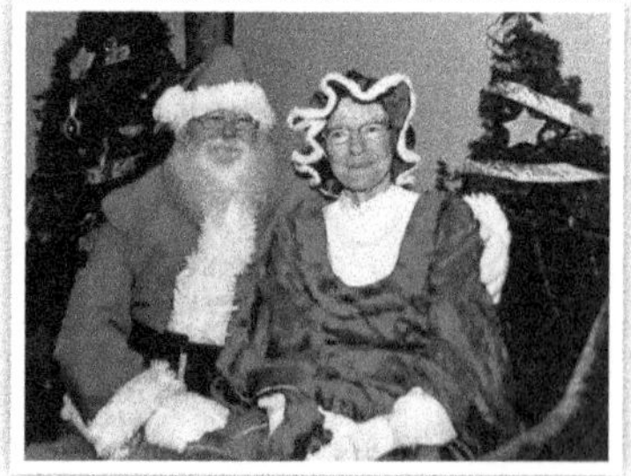

As mentioned earlier, I had to quit posing as Santa because of the confusion it presented for Beth. It was a part of a life that I will always treasure and remember fondly but no longer to be.

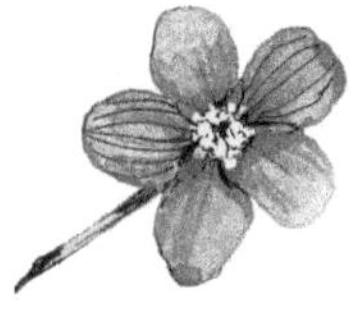

Chapter: Year 3

JAN 21, 2013

Trip to Edmonton to see the only neurologist that was available, a young lady that had just finished her degree; it went as if we were her first patient. Basically, all that happened was the same assessment that was conducted back at our GP with one exception…she used the words "Dementia"!! Oh shit!!! This was the first time this word was mentioned with Beth present; not good! Dementia is a broad term for what was happening, and she added there was a potential for Alzheimer's; double 'Oh Shit!!!' Tried to get more specific information on the disease, and what to expect; however, there was nothing to ease the shock and provide any hope. We were scheduled for another appointment, and another assessment. The drive home was very subdued.

MAY 16, 2013

In light of the assessment, and with fragile discussions with Beth, we determined that we had to get our affairs in order; something that should have been done years ago. At this stage, Beth is still lucid and understanding of the importance of this action; still not something I take pleasure in. It is;

however, the determination of the lawyer that Beth is capable of making these decisions on her own behalf, and the necessary documentation was legalized.

JUNE, 2013

Driving is now becoming an issue which is causing real concern. I feel that I can't trust her ability to drive anymore, especially on her own. While arriving at the A&W in Rimbey, she was cutting corners and clipped a few curbs in the parking lot. The worst part is that she gets really upset If I even suggest a correction to her driving methods. This is where I feel responsible, and don't know what to do. Is it my fault that she can't function because I don't let her keep in practice, or is my fear founded? She used to be a great driver, and now it's getting quite scary.

It has been brought up many times in the recent past, by family members, where concern was voiced regarding her ability to drive. Till now, I have always kept a real close eye on her driving, and don't let her drive-in high traffic areas.

We attended a seminar of sorts… more like a protest, where seniors were upset with the concept of losing their driving licenses. It was sponsored by AMA, I think, and was attended by government officials, police, and the medical profession; the latter are put to task to advise patients of the requirement to lose licenses. The protest was as violent and boisterous as a bunch of seniors, sitting down, could be… a horrific sight indeed, police were blocked from eating doughnuts!! Being silly of course!

In reality, many were upset at the concept; nevertheless, the issue of people with dementia was raised, and it didn't go over well with Beth. Driving from that point on was vastly more restricted and eventually was eliminated altogether. My reasoning for mentioning this, is the potential for a lot of anxiety over this issue; something to consider well in advance.

10 JULY, 2013 NEUROLOGIST EDMONTON

Our second appointment with the neurologist in Edmonton. With this appointment she confirmed "Alzheimer's"! Finally, an official confirmation of a potential diagnosis of Alzheimer's! I know… clear as mud!! Remember, they can't confirm the certainty until an autopsy is performed; however, ratification was a long time coming. Had to see a neurologist to find out what I already knew by now. Beth was again quiet; nonetheless, seemed to accept the prognosis.

Went back at the GP and he prescribed 'Aricept', a common drug used for Alzheimer's. And now it begins! I mentioned that I was less than pleased with the neurologist, and suggested that I wanted a second opinion, not because I doubted the diagnosis, because there was little useful information regarding diagnosis, processes, and expectations, so he set up another appointment with a neurology specialist.

SEPT 25, 2013

Understanding, empathy, and patience are the key attitudes of the day… always!! It is becoming very difficult to hold any form of discussion, points of view, debate, and even joking around. Now the flavour of the day consists solely of basic instructions, positive thoughts, and carefully thought-out words; no more back tracking or excuses.

Explanations must be well thought out and simple, instructions of any sort are not fully understood! I must keep my guard up all the time, it's hard to change my personality traits, and it's an ongoing process; nonetheless, I will learn as it does make the day go by more easily.

NOV 27, 2013

Things are proceeding quite well with Beth, although she seems to be having increased confusion. Hard to explain! Went to Edmonton yesterday because we had a dentist appointment for my dad. Coming home, Beth needed to eat, so I suggested Timmy's. "No", so then suggested Subway. When we got there, she said, "I thought we were going to Timmy's", etc.

Day before, it was the same with going to Sears, or not, finally went to Sears, and she bought two nice blouses. She needs someone that can shop with her and talk styles. She gets frustrated with me going off to the Hardware area, then coming back, as she then feels rushed. I've tried staying with her and encouraging her to try things on, yet, she declines as it seems to pressure her.

28 NOV, 2013

We resigned from the Rimbey Lions Club today because Beth didn't want to go to the meetings. She wanted me to go by myself; however, there's no way I would leave her alone. They were very understanding, without specifically knowing why we are quitting; I think they suspected what is happening based on their response. Again, the hardest issue right now is for Beth to let people know what is going on. She doesn't want any form of pity (for lack of a better word), or the reactions people have. "How are you feeling?" "Is there anything I can do?" "I understand what you're going through", etc.

DEC 3, 2013

Watched a Documentary by David Suzuki regarding his mother's Alzheimer's; good video if you can find it. It took a while to understand what it was about, but I stuck with it and it was worthwhile.

The biggest issue I can see right now is not having a support network. In our current situation is not necessarily for me to find support, it's extremely hard for me to attend. I can't leave Beth alone, and she doesn't want to associate with any other individuals or groups, especially on her own.

We had a moment of acceptance yesterday. I mentioned getting rid of one car, and Beth burst into tears and said, "I've lost half of my life!" Caught me off guard and I asked what she meant. She said, "I used to drive!" We shed a few tears together and discussed that she couldn't drive because of her eyesight (she sees double when looking at vehicles), and she accepted it. All in all, it went pretty well; we agreed to enjoy life as it comes. We have been having fun together, and I am trying to do the things she wants, as much as she wants. She does enjoy going to the Wooden Shoe for breakfasts, so we go frequently. Lately she loves her "pie & ice cream" in the afternoon. It's all good.

DEC 23, 2013

Beth is doing OK. At times she seems quite feisty, and that is what I/we have fun with. I play on it to bring out her sense of humour and smiles.

I've been working on a routine that seems to work. Going to Wooden Shoe for Breakfast in the morning, and around 3:00 p.m. we go to Subway for a lunch break. It's relatively cheap and gives her an outing, especially when there is nothing she can do to help me around the house. I know we should eat at home; nonetheless, I do most of the cooking and it gives me a break. We do cook a major meal for supper.

The confusion seems to be increasing lately. I think the stress of Christmas is affecting her. She is constantly concerned about what we are doing, when we are doing it, and who is getting what, etc. She confuses my sister's party with going to our son's place. She is constantly concerned about what everybody is getting for gifts. She'll see something, and decide she needs to get it for someone, so they'll have a gift to open; not a problem as they're small gifts.

DEC 24, 2013

Well Christmas is upon us, and we had planned well in advance to go to my sister's place to have a Christmas get together with family, especially for dad. We were to return home, then leaving again to go to George's to stay overnight, spend Christmas with them, stay overnight again, then come back home.

Went through a lot of aggravation with Beth. She woke up saying she wasn't going because she wasn't feeling good. I know she has a bit of a cold, and she didn't look good, yet I'll have to admit I thought she just was making excuses. I was visibly upset; nevertheless, did cancel the Oil Change appointment, and called my sister and our son to tell them we weren't going. Let Beth go back to sleep for a couple hour; when she got up, she decided to go, I didn't pressure her, and we packed up and went.

The visit was OK for the most part; however, it didn't go well when we got home. There was anxiety for Christmas Day, and the trip to our son's place. First it was "we're not going anywhere", then "when are they getting here", then "why didn't you tell me we we're supposed to go there", then "why didn't we stay there tonight", then "why do you get upset all the time?". There definitely was no arguing, all I did was tell her the facts, it doesn't matter what I say, it just doesn't register. Can't make plans, nor commitments anymore.

DEC 25, 2013

This is the worst Christmas of my life. Christ gave me a shit load of Hell for Christmas! When the Almighty dumps on you on his Birthday, it's hard to have any faith or hope. I am crying my eyes out this morning while Beth is sleeping in anticipation of what today will bring. Last night pretty much ended up in discord, and with staying home today. I'm going to go with "Yes Dear", "OK", "Sure", "Good idea", and "I Love you Hon!".

Well, OK, there is a God, and he will help when in need. When Beth got up, I went with as said. I also got a divine inspiration from above. I text Amanda with words "Phone with no pressure". She caught on, and phoned Beth to asked if we were going to visit. It's almost like Beth's eyes lit up with excitement and agreed to go. Turned out to be a great visit for Christmas day which extended even after we came home Christmas night.

DEC 27, 2013

I've always been the proponent of giving Beth an equal voice. Our married life has consisted of the "What would you like to do?", "No, what would YOU like to do???" game. It's hard to break old habits. I've never been the 'my way or the highway' type; 'Equal partners, equal voice' so to speak. I am trying to learn what works, and it seems that collaborating on a decision and making plans together doesn't.

Deciding we were going to our son's while at my sister's place on the 24th, might have resulted in frustration the next day when I would tell her what we agreed to do the night before. The stress comes in when I had to phone our son to tell him we were not coming. I wouldn't be able to say, "Beth doesn't want to go", or "Beth changed her mind", she would then get mad that I'm blaming her. As such I must sometimes lie to my family and friends about breaking plans, and that it may happen time and again, at the spur of the moment.

DEC 31, 2013

Beth is starting to get upset watching movies with any form of violence. I've noticed it in the last month or so. If we watch anything like RED, Walking Dead, or Kungfu Charlie, etc. before going to bed, she has a restless night. As such I've switched to watching Old Classics as the last show before going to bed, and it seems to work. It's an on/off thing; she doesn't object to some shows, so I watch carefully, and if she gets antsy, I just change to a different show midway through. We must have seen a hundred Christmas movies lately.

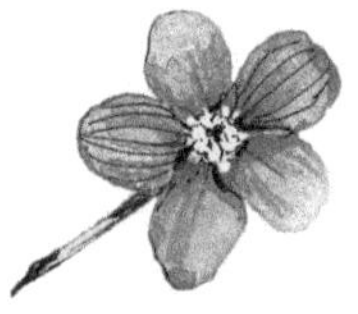

Chapter: Year 4

FEB 4, 2014

Well, we have some new learnings, and some new complications.

COMPLICATIONS

Beth is now potentially diagnosed with an Autonomous Thyroid which, I guess, means that her Thyroid isn't working as it should. Thought this could be the reason for her weight loss but according to tests done by our GP, her Thyroid was working fine till about six months ago. The specialist keeps asking if she is "shaking", and yes, there is a bit of shakiness that I've noticed. He's trying something like a kick-start with some medication to see if it helps, and she will be doing blood work every month to keep track of progress.

NEW LEARNINGS

Lately I've noticed Beth is having trouble with numbers. There are two aspects of this, first is that Beth can't drive anymore, and I know it drives her nuts. As mentioned before, she tends to see double vehicles, sometimes she sees people where there are none…like "three people sitting in the ditch" … in wintertime.

The other aspect is with preparing things to eat. Beth tends to set places for three instead of just the two of us. There's always an extra plate, knife, or fork. She asked if I wanted some chocolate almonds the other day, and showed up with two bowls…then went back for hers. I try to explain that there are only two of us, sometimes she includes someone we just saw on TV. I'm learning to just accept, and not question her on it.

There are also issues with taking care of her that really have me going; she got really upset at me for taking care of her at night. We woke up at 3:30 a.m., and I asked her how she was doing, to which she responded that she was cold. I explained that the heat blanket was on, and she uncovers herself because she gets too warm. In the morning all hell broke loose, "What gives you the right to come in my room and spy on me?" WTF? Tried to explain that it's our room, we sleep together, and that I was just trying to take care of her. She says she's, "grown up and can take care of herself". I'm finding that it's impossible and futile to defend myself, even when I'm right. Seems like I just have to take care of the issue, and not talk about it.

19 FEBRUARY, 2014

Went to Edmonton to see a neurology specialist, needed a professional second opinion. The appointment went quite well, the three of us spent a lot of time together, then we were analysed separately. When we got back together the diagnosis of Alzheimer's was again confirmed. I'm not sure what type of Alzheimer's he identified; however, I'm pretty sure it was frontal lobe. Again, my mind was suffering pure distress, and I wasn't able to capture the essence of the prognosis. He was rather candid regarding the diagnosis, and rightfully so, by then Beth had joined us, and it would have caused her a lot of stress. She was reserved as it was. My poor Beth! I'm at a loss, what can I do???

MAR 12, 2014

Throughout this stage of Beth's life, she has dramatically lost a lot of weight. Went from an estimation of 170 lbs to 115 lbs, seemingly overnight. We finally got a diagnosis of a hyperactive Thyroid. What happened next is unexplainable as described in the following excerpts from my letter to Beth's neurologist!!

You saw Dorothy (Beth) Blais on the nineteenth of February, and provided a diagnosis of Alzheimer's. There is an incident of relevance to which you should become aware.

On the eighth of January, Beth saw a doctor with respect to a Thyroid condition that may have resulted in Beth losing weight. The doctor prescribed Pms-Metoprolol-L (Metoprolol Tartrate) to bring down a high heart rate, and a Thyroid Uptake and scan for the thirtieth and thirty-first of January. The results of the Thyroid Uptake were confirmation of an overactive Thyroid.

The doctor then scheduled Beth to have a Radioactive Iodine (RAI) Thyroid Treatment on the twenty-first of February, and prescribed Tapazole (Methimazole) for Beth to begin immediately after the RAI treatment for her Thyroid condition, continuing for two weeks afterwards. She was instructed to quit taking the Bata Blocker for that duration as well.

The reason for this email is what appears to be the effects the procedure had on Beth. About the time the medication was finished, I noticed that Beth was extremely cognitive, and full of energy. No one would have even suspected Beth had Alzheimer's. She started doing things I used to have to do for her, she even cooked a couple meals. Now that it's been almost three weeks after the medication, it seems she is starting to revert to conditions prior to the treatment or mediation.

This raises many questions from a layman's point of view: Could one of, or a combination of, medications have provided the clarity of mind? Could this be a potential treatment for Alzheimer's? Could the RAI treatment have caused this effect? Could part of the problem be her Thyroid?

Never got an answer!

12 MAY, 2014

I wrote previously regarding my foray into the 'Santa Zone', where Beth and I entertained children around the Rimbey area, something we had to give up two years ago. My perfectly white beard, combined with my 'elfish stature', my girth, and button nose, made me a natural for the part. Well as things have a propensity to do, they had to change!!!

Big day for me today, I must go in for an operation, and subsequently, I was instructed to shave my beard of thirty-nine years. It occurred to me that I don't think Beth had ever seen me without a beard.

Because of Beth's current state of confusion, and to lessen any future stress, I was worried Beth would consider me a stranger if I just suddenly appeared in her world sans beard. When the time came that I had to shave, I brought her into the bathroom, and together, with both of our hands on the hair trimmer, we began the process. It worked out perfectly, and although I'll never know if it was an issue later in the journey, there was never any confusion of whom I was that I could perceive.

Perhaps something for you to think about regarding any change of appearance. It is hard enough on a confused mind to not have to deal with these kinds of surprises.

In the ongoing saga of my beard, it has been brought to my attention that I resemble my father, an honour I relish greatly. So, I don't know if I will grow my beard back or not in the near nor distant future.

25 MAY, 2014

I am starting to notice problems with asking her to help me decide on anything. I've always been the type to ask, "Where should we go eat?", "What are you hungry for?", "What do you want to do?", now, that never works. I find that I must make suggestions, and ask for her opinion; however, even that doesn't work all the time. It seems that telling her what I feel like eating, what I want to do, or where I need to go works best. Problem is, I'm not the pushy type, and I have always tried to get feedback and make consensual decisions. It's been the foundation of our relationship, and now it makes me feel like I alone make the decisions (bossy, controlling). That's hard for a "wishy-washy" person to do.

JUNE 2014

At this juncture I thought it prudent to provide some dos and don'ts for effective communication.

DON'T

1. Don't try to reason - their mind is undisputable;
2. Don't argue - you cannot win;
3. Don't confront - invokes the 'Fight' response as they cannot 'Flight';
4. Don't remind them what they forget - you are introducing something new into their lives;
5. Don't question recent memory loss - same as above;
6. Don't take it personally - you are now a caregiver, no longer a spouse.

DO

1. Give short, one sentence explanations;
2. Allow plenty of time for comprehension… then triple it;
3. Repeat instructions, in sentences, in exactly the same way;
4. Eliminate "but" from your vocabulary, substitute "still";
5. Avoid insistence – try again later;
6. Agree with them or distract them to a different subject or activity;
7. Accept the blame when something's wrong, especially if you're right;
8. Gracefully leave the room, if necessary, to avoid confrontations;
9. Respond to the feelings rather than the words;
10. Be patient, cheerful, and reassuring;
11. Go with the flow;
12. Practice 100% forgiveness.

JULY 2014

Her observation is quite acute regardless of her comprehension. Cooking is getting scary now because she sometimes loses a grasp of how the burner controls work. Just to explain, we finished cooking the other day, and she was upset because all the burners were not all pointing up, the temperature dial for the oven was set at 350 Celsius even though we weren't cooking anything, and the oven was turned off… I turned the dial to zero Celsius. I try to keep her involved, yet it is becoming a concern if I get her to help me cook.

The other day she called me to the basement because she couldn't figure out the difference between the washer and dryer, and how to get them to work. Again, I seem to be taking over all the functions, and I can't expect her do anything on her own. A minor setback…now, do I separate the whites or the colours?? And what about this 'Bleach' stuff??

SEPT 12, 2014

Lately, things have been going relatively well. Latest observations are that instructions, reasoning, and discussions are strained. When Beth makes up her mind there is little chance of changing it. Basically, what she wants she gets. Discussing things in public will not happen as Beth feels we are arguing, and she gets angry quickly. In public, any conversation is a whisper as she feels everyone can hear, and is listening.

Another observation is that any future commitment is a real issue, and she will avoid it as much as possible. When appointments or commitments are made, timing becomes an issue as she has no concept of when the appointment is, when to get ready, and when we have to leave. Beth will start to prepare for guests' days in advance with the thought that the upcoming visit is imminent. I still haven't learned!!!

OCT 9, 2014

Lots has been happening. A dearly beloved uncle of mine passed away from Alzheimer's on Oct 1st. Went to BC for his Celebration of Life. It was great to reunite, and visit with my aunt and my cousins, hadn't seen them in quite a while. This family is so special because Uncle Phil was a consummate jokester comedian, and the apples didn't fall far from the tree.

Though the occasion was solemn, the wake was befitting the Irish… which they weren't. Unfortunately, Beth found the laughing and revelry quite overwhelming. She doesn't do good in a crowd with lots of conversations going on, especially if the voice volume is raised through laughter or comradery. She was concerned about them taking all our money, and was disturbed about the subject matter of many of the conversations that were taking place. Will try to keep associations to smaller crowds from now on.

NOV 20, 2014

Beth is regressing quite a bit, although still manageable. She has a problem with the words "let's go to bed". Lately, when I say that, she changes from her PJs, puts on her jeans and shoes, and is ready to go somewhere. "let's go" to her must mean "hop in the car" to go somewhere. I can't figure out where "bed" is. It's basically been like this for three nights now.

Time, as a concept just doesn't relate, "going to Edmonton tomorrow" means getting dressed for travel right now. She tries to remember appointments, then, when I say we have an appointment to go to, she gets upset because "I didn't tell her".

Yesterday, my jeans were in the wash, and I needed a pair of pants to go out. When I tried on an old pair of jeans, that I couldn't buckle up any longer, she got upset because I wouldn't try on some shirts she pulled out for me. She got upset that I wouldn't even try them on. The concept of shirts verses pants was lost on her. I couldn't reason that I needed a pair of pants, and not a shirt. I even tried putting my legs in a sweater to show her it doesn't work. Next time, I will try on the shirts ***as a shirt*** to see what she says or does.

Also, her speech composition is waning quite a bit. It's getting extremely hard to understand Beth, yet, I can usually establish what she is trying to say. At least she tries to communicate, it's far better than having her just clam up. I really think being on the road a lot is helpful! She opens up and talks to me, usually about seeing something, or some memory. Sometimes she surprises me by recalling things I have forgotten.

We do have a lot of hugs and kisses going on. I can tell she appreciates me being there, and admits to needing me, even to other people.

DEC 3, 2014

I guess I'll never learn, giving her choices are hard for her. Asked her if she wanted to plate the fried veggies, or put them in a Corning Ware bowl (to keep warm in the oven) so we could fry ham in the same fry pan? Answer was, "No, because the Corning Ware would cool off the veggies". Reinforcing the original question just upset her; ended up warming the Corning Ware bowl in oven, then putting veggies in, and keeping them heated in oven. Point is to only ask once, then listen carefully; although, mostly better to just decide, and not ask. She was right about veggies cooling off, plating would have been the wrong thing to do.

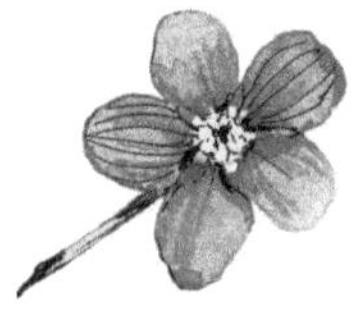

Chapter: Year 5

JAN 22, 2015

New developments.

Beth has started having a problem with dressing herself. She now asks, and allows me to help her. This is great because with the confusion she would spend a lot of time trying to figure out what to wear. I'm finding more and more that, letting her do things her way until she asks, is increasing her self-esteem. Results are usually quite good.

We still enjoy going for rides together, be it for shopping, lunch, or just plain sightseeing. Occasionally she keeps suggesting she wants us to go East, I'm assuming to Saskatchewan. I interpret this as wanting to escape, and go on a trip. It could just stem from seeing Corner Gas the Movie which is set in Saskatchewan; plan to make a trip there in the spring

FEB 1, 2015

Important observation: in every relationship existing, you will experience moments of frustration, anxiety, depression, anger, resulting from a disagreement of sorts; that can't happen with Alzheimer's!!!

I needed to use the snowblower yesterday, and Beth wanted to help me. *(OMG, I can't remember how to spell "ove"(of)).* She said she could help push it or turn the discharge crank. Of course, for safety reasons I considered this as out of the question. Had a hard time explaining that there was nothing she could do to help me. She resisted any suggestions to clear snow from the porch. Once the job was completed, Beth seemed reserved and sad.

In hindsight, It occurred to me that perhaps she just wanted to be with me, and do things together as we used to do. Something to think about, as this is now fodder for remorse. If it were only possible to let her help me now!!! In reality, it wouldn't have been a bad idea to just go slowly, carefully, and let her help. Hell, the snow wasn't going anywhere, and neither were we. Think about it, her mind is feeling anxiety, and emotions as much as yours. Capture any opportunity to connect with and unite as one again as those opportunities present themselves.

It is impossible to expect her to do anything on her own. She is very attached to me, and doesn't want me to be out of her sight. I'm OK with that, in fact, I love it! We've never been closer, and I know it might be a potential problem later when she must be placed in a care facility; nevertheless, I'm revelling in the moment.

CONSEQUENCES

With the realization that Beth does not want to be separated from me at any time, one of my biggest concerns right now is, 'what if something happens to me?' A broken leg or even just the flu could be a catastrophe.

There is no situation in the world that you can rationalize that will become an acceptable solution for you, or your spouse, if you are incapacitated! You might have access to neighbours, friends, or relatives that are more than willing to step in, nevertheless, they will never fulfill your requirement for the level of care and support you want to provide; she is yours, and that is it! Furthermore, with the attachment she has formed, absence due to hospitalization would be a substantial burden.

Everything revealed so far pertains mainly to your wellbeing; however, it also applies to her physical and psychological wellbeing as well. What happens if she is the one that breaks a leg, or worse, a hip? Can you imagine the confusion and frustration with her having to deal with a situation she is not the least familiar with?

Regardless of whom becomes disabled, there are some pitfalls with any type of casualty! You must consider how any situation will impact her, and more so, how will she respond to any of those situations? Should something befall you, how will anyone else tasked with her care respond to any situation? "Hey son, take care of your mom while I lay in the hospital for a couple weeks". These factors should be a major consideration before you take up mountain climbing or any other extreme activity.

To exemplify the importance of mobility, I don't condone drinking and driving, and once responsibility entered my life, I became very concerned with consumption, and the prospect of having to drive home. I can't stress enough the importance of not drinking and driving!!

We used to relax at home, and after dinner would enjoy a drink or three of anything on hand; once Beth was diagnosed with Cancer, back in 2011, both Beth and I quit drinking cold Turkey; I mean nothing at all! I won't even have a glass of wine or a beer while out for dinner or visiting friends, in case we get pulled over, and there is even the scent of alcohol on my breath. We live on an acreage close to Gull Lake, Northwest of Red Deer, Alberta. The closest Village to us is Rimbey to the West, or Bentley to the South, both 13 KMs away. If I would ever get my license revoked, for any reason, we would be, literally, thumbing our way around, and at this stage of Beth's life, that would be unimaginable and impossible!!

11 FEB, 2015

Really had a hard night last night! We are going to go for supper with my dad on Sunday the 15th, Beth was concerned about getting ready (dressed), and about people coming over. I reassured her we weren't going anywhere tonight at least five times. I managed to stay calm and reassuring; however, this time she got really upset with me for not telling her what was happening; she felt I was keeping things from her. Couldn't get it out of her mind that we weren't going right now or in a few minutes or even tonight, and that no one was coming to our place. She seems to be developing anxiety and some form of aggression out of confusion and frustration. I believe the perception of time is absent, anything said is current in her mind.

It's hard to have any form of conversation without mentioning, or discussing, a plan for some time in the future, and I must learn to live in the present, and not forecast any event.

15 APRIL, 2015

Beth is showing a lot of confusion regarding getting dressed, most specifically, changing shoes. She will take one off, and put another shoe on, then gets confused as to what to do next. She'll take the other one off then put it back on. Sometimes she'll match different shoes, left with left and right with right, and then gets stumped on which goes with which. She also has a hard time associating which shoes are for what…outdoor hikers vs indoor slippers.

25 MAY, 2015

Feeling depressed and overwhelmed tonight. Like the last couple nights, I wake up at 1:30 a.m., and can't sleep till 5:00 a.m. We're going camping to Sir Winston Churchill Provincial Park today; this should be interesting! I'm exhausted and stressed out to the max working on four hrs sleep a night. I get to the point where I'm ready to collapse by 3:00 p.m., yet, if I try to get some shut eye on the couch, Beth immediately gets up, and starts doing something on her own, and that's not good.

Don't know how to post this; however, I'm starting to see where my frustration sets in. It seems that when things are important to me, like handling the requirements to get everything ready, I don't have or make time to address Beth's issues. She wants to go; however, wants to bring or do weird things prior to leaving, and I just don't seem to have time for it. I need to allow her needs to evolve into requirements that suit the issue at hand, rather than just saying "we can't do or bring that", and hope it dies a natural death.

I can see that I must make her needs a priority rather than mine. Need a lot more prep time!

Pissed off about all the fundraising going on for Cancer, MS, etc., and yet, almost nothing for Alzheimer's; and I now realize why. There is an Alzheimer's fundraising walk occurring; however, close family members involved in caregiving for an Alzheimer's patient, don't have time or ability to do any fundraising; thereby, the fundraising is poorly attended, and research doesn't get funded. If the money collected for even one Cancer fundraising event were channeled to Alzheimer's, a cure could be found within a year.

I don't want to sound crass, still, just to make my point, close family of Cancer patients mostly feel anger, sympathy, and empathy; conversely, Alzheimer's caregivers are also stretched and stressed to the limit, as they try to comprehend what is happening, and how to cope and handle most situations; there are no instructions! All the while, they realize a hopeless prognosis, and the imminent end results, if you will. Funny thing about this disease is that, though the patient is not suffering the pain and agony of the other diseases, the patient doesn't even realize they have an issue. They just can't figure out why you're acting so weird.

At least with Cancer there is hope! Many Cancer patients can now be cured or have a life extension of sorts, not one Alzheimer's patient can!

13 JUNE, 2015

Before I give you a shot of reality, there is one more aspect regarding your health you must consider. The trials and tribulations you are about to experience in the care of your spouse with Alzheimer's, is akin to an extreme sport that you don't want to partake in; unfortunately, at this point you don't have a choice! No, it won't break your leg, at least not directly; however, it will play havoc with your brain. The downside is that your psychological wellbeing will suffer; trust me on this one. It will test your metal to the breaking point; for me, it was depression! When you are tasked to the care of someone you love, cherish, and wish the best for; you cannot afford to let your caregiving waver. I survived, as you will, and in the process, you will hopefully become a stronger, humbler person.

And now for the long story. Had a bout of depression Monday morning. We were to see dad Tuesday, and when I woke up at 1:30 in the morning, my mind went nuts (disturbed), and couldn't sleep till 6:30 a.m. Don't worry, nothing suicidal, I don't have those tendencies or even thoughts, and I've been through depression before.

The depression started about a month ago centred around a weird image I saw, and couldn't comprehend, on a Health Supplement advertisement regarding a 'Miracle Diabetes Cure made from Kelp'. I listened to the complete presentation, which lasted a complete half hour yet, nowhere was there any recurrence, nor mention of this image. This image kept bugging me!! The image showed someone with indentations on (her) knees, or for some time I thought they might have been two fingers, with some green balls still stuck to a few of the indentations. Couldn't figure out how that could be related to Diabetes, and Tuesday, it came to a head; along with an explosion of weird mind-boggling thoughts that I could not find a resolve for; everything seemed hopeless. Sort of like a song you heard, don't know the title of, don't know the singer, and don't know the words to, and yet you can't get out of your mind.

I did a google search, and when I keyed in "Kneeling on" it came up with "Kneeling on frozen peas", and there was my image, along with an explanation of it as being a form of school punishment. At least I had an explanation, yet it still didn't resolve my anxiety. By the way, attached to the site there were more "Freaky" images that seemed to defy explanation to me, and created a lot of "F" words…a Freak show of sorts, and mostly photoshopped, as I found out. Don't explore any further, I don't want to blow your mind as well.

Anyways, I finally did fall asleep for a couple hours, and then got a hold of my sister. She's a wonder!! She explained how my mind was working, and it makes perfect sense under my circumstances.

Saw the Doc on Tuesday, and I am now on anti-depressants and sleeping pills. Tuesday night I had the most wonderful sleep I've had in years. Went to bed at 11:30 p.m., and fell right back asleep, after waking up three times for Beth, till the phone rang at 11:30 a.m. Felt great all day. As I mentioned, I'm now on anti-depressants, sleeping pills, and going to see a Counselor soon as it can be arranged.

5 JULY, 2015

Busy month, we finally met our Grand Niece. What a perfect little Angel!!! We met up with my cousin and her daughter from BC, and took them to see dad. We went to my sister's place for supper, as before, Beth got more and more agitated because of the crowds.

On the sixth, I promised her that when this was over, we would head out for Saskatchewan to see the Corner Gas series set. You should have seen the look on her face, like a twelve-year-old being told they were going to Disney Land for the first time. On the eight we left to fulfill my promise of 22 Jan, 2015.

We were supposed to go to our Grand Niece's Baptism on the seventh; however, Beth was not faring well so decided against it. She slept until 11:30 a.m.

8 JULY, 2015

As promised, left for Saskatchewan to see one of our most treasured destinations, mine at least. Beth was excited to hit the road, and all went well; that is until time for lunch, and a restroom break. Reason I mention this is that lunch went OK, the bathroom break… not so much. I continually keep a very close eye on Beth; however, an incident occurred that had me bewildered.

I was in the lineup for our food order at the Gas Station Subway (not sure where this was), and had full view of the washroom doors. When Beth rejoined me, she was obviously disturbed; she related that some man was in the bathroom using a mop. Couldn't understand what she was talking about as I was sure this couldn't have happened. I wasn't watching the doorway 100% of the time; however, I saw no one enter or leave the facilities except Beth.

Her story didn't seem plausible, and I thought maybe just a bit of delusion, not knowing what to expect with Alzheimer's, anything is possible; maybe this was something new to watch for. Surely if any man would have walked into an occupied lady's washroom, he would have apologized, and excused himself. My only thought was that she went into a storage room when a person from a clean-up crew was there, and yet, I should have noticed that happening.

Don't know what went on; wasn't sure if she even used the facilities, although she was gone for an appropriate amount of time. Said she was OK, and didn't have to go anymore; got our order and left.

The trip was OK for the most part except, more and more, Beth doesn't travel well. The traveling part is OK, nonetheless, she obviously has a lot of anxiety regarding washrooms. She is always concerned regarding someone using it even if it has multiple stalls.

Campsite washrooms are especially becoming a bust as well, regardless of how clean they are. She says she won't use them because there are little kids around, even when there aren't any. I don't know if she worries about the noise or the mess they make, or just her shyness. She might feel people will walk in on her.

Don't know what to do; the Westphalia might have to go! Might try to find an older motor home with a bathroom or might have to just 'Motel it' for trips. (YUCK!)

26 JULY, 2015

Uncle Tom went into the hospital yesterday, diagnosed with Pancreatic Cancer. Such an interesting character; he was one of the last of a dying breed of cowboys. Always wore cowboy hat and boots, and always drove huge cars like Lincolns or Cadillacs. He always disliked, and was vocal of anything to do with the government. He expressed himself as opinionated, hard-nosed, and with a boisterous voice and laughter. Not the kind of man the meek and mild take to; however, he was a pussycat, always entertaining, and I loved the guy.

Funny, this depression thing! While in Edmonton we went to see Nan's grave. Had a bout of depression in that I realized that with dad, Uncle Tom, and Beth's conditions, that things are never going to get better. I was depressed for about 5 minutes then realized that if things were never going to get better, then this is as good as it's going to get… so… enjoy and treasure each moment, before it does get worse. Must be the pills talking; nonetheless, it works for me! Savoring every moment!

27 JULY, 2015

Today, Beth just had another RAI Treatment for her Thyroid. She is on medication for post RAI Treatment again, and I am watching closely for the same side effects as her last treatment of Feb 2014 (Ref: Mar 12, 2014) …it didn't happen.

She needs more and more help daily, which is a pleasure to do. Spending quality time with her is very important to me now. She clings to me very closely, and asks me to be with her as if she would be expected to "go it alone." I reassure her that I'm always going to be with her, as I want to be. I cannot bear to see the fear in her eyes, as a reflection of the devastation she would feel if I ever left her, which of course would never happen. I see and feel the fear she must be going through as we progress through this damned disease.

I wish I could make someone understand the desperation I feel regarding the fundraising efforts in place for cancer, MS, diabetes, heart disease, and yet, so little for Alzheimer's; it still disturbs me.

1 AUG, 2015

Sad day! Uncle Tom passed away today! His sister (Beth's mom) lives in Calgary, he had no children, and his wife preceded his passing by quite some time. Beth and I were pretty much the closest people to him; both physically and mentally. Because of Beth's Alzheimer's, I became Executor by default; I was put to task to make his arrangements.

He didn't have any finances to speak of, and had never prepared for this event, as it mattered little to him. His idea was to just "throw his ashes out someplace". On his death bed, he did tell me to just spread his ashes on Nan's grave; something that is frowned upon. Out of true respect for the man, and through many legal concerns, I was able to arrange having his urn placed in Nan's grave site, just above her casket. There is no tombstone or place-marker of any kind for him; nonetheless, something I know they both would appreciate.

There are so many things to add stress into your life, especially when you are deeply attached to taking care of your loved one during this turbulent time in her ordeal. It wasn't a pleasant task, yet I felt so privileged to do so. I found the diversion of handling Uncle Tom's arrangements a welcomed relief from the everyday stress I have been subject to lately.

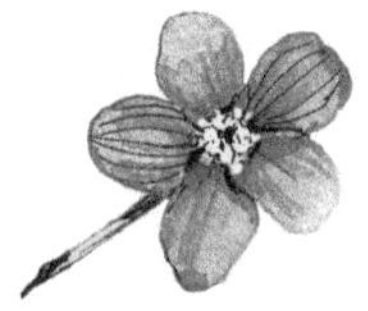

Chapter: The Contempt of Familiarity

Contempt: definition is - the act of despising.

Of course, this is a play on words of the popular saying "Familiarity Breeds Contempt", which refers to the fact that when things are constant, you get bored with the redundancy, and tend to want a change; subsequently, you begin to despise the familiarity. I am referring to the contempt of the familiarity of seeing my precious Beth struggling with the constant confusion Alzheimer's is imposing on her life; something I perceive, and must adjust for, or accommodate, on a daily basis.

Interesting incident, in typing the heading for this chapter, my finger missed the 'm' and hit the 'n'. A common mistake; nonetheless, this time with an amazing consequence; spellcheck came up with the 'Content of Familiarity', the total opposite of my intended demeanour. It took a while to sink in, it did; however, make me think about my situation. Throughout my time with Beth, the familiarity we shared was filled with nothing but content. Even to this day, I would not change a moment I had with Beth, and would gladly do it all again, even knowing the inevitable outcome. As such, both sayings hold true!!

24 SEPT, 2015

Figured it was time to review and recap thoughts of the current situation.

Beth continues to be deteriorating as time seems to move quickly by… at a snail's pace! Things are going OK, and I don't see the decline as much as others do. I am reminded; however, of how fast time is passing by, as I refill the pill box every Sunday; weeks fly by! As far as changes, there are not many that are radical to the point that I can say, "And now she can no longer do…", it just doesn't work that way.

Sometimes she will slip into a temporary lapse where she doesn't know what door of the car to get into, or how to find her seat belt. Sometimes she won't know how to open the door from the inside. She will pull the handle, and yet, not push outward on the door; then she will know how to open the door for the next two weeks (of course, this occurrence is subjective as to time passage; however, that pretty much nails it down).

Most things she can do quite well on her own with a little prodding from me. Getting dressed for bed can be confusing, especially if we have someplace to go the next day. She has a hard time relating time lapses. As an example, if reminded we are going to go to someone's birthday in four days, she will think we have to get ready and dress for the occasion today, or even when going to bed, etc. It doesn't happen all the time; however, I must tell her repeatedly that we have lots of time, we're not going right now, today, tonight, or even tomorrow.

Her speech is the hardest hurdle right now. When in public, especially in restaurants, she talks in a whisper so no one can hear us. Unfortunately, with the ambient noise, and teeny-bopper type music of today, neither can I.

Ordering food is an issue as we usually get rushed, and I can't nail down what she would like to eat. She jumps from menu item to menu item, and when it comes time to order, will usually order what I do. We do like the same things, so it's not usually an issue.

It's hard for her to relay what she wants to say at the best of time. She substitutes nonrelated, yet similar words, into her conversation. Hard to explain that one, something like "open the window meaning open the door", "leave the door open meaning leave the light on?", I do catch on however. The latest one is saying yes, and meaning no, which is becoming more prevalent. That's a hard one to rationalize, as I'm never sure what she means, or wants to do… must figure out a way to ask the question differently…it will come.

Shopping can be a drudgery, and yet, sometimes fun. Yesterday, in Edmonton, she spotted a Wholesale Sports Store, and wanted to go in. Usually that involves lots of money, and a return trip to return purchases the next day; quite enjoyable actually.

This time it was just a look-see. I have been looking for a PJ top for a while now, and that, she is aware of. While looking, we ran across some long sleeve camo style sweatshirts that I guess could be used for that purpose. Saw two that were on the same rack, almost side by side, and were almost identical in design, just a different camo pattern on them. Showed them both to Beth, and said these could work. She picked one, and I said I liked the other… then I showed her the price…hers was $149.99, and mine was $24.59. I said, jokingly, "I knew you would pick that one, you have expensive tastes!". She chuckled and smiled…we moved on. See, it's not all bad, we do have fun.

She wants to help do things. She wanted me to teach here how to use tools so she could help build our projects. That is an impossibility at this juncture as she cannot grasp any instructions whatsoever; if the hammer is between a knife and a fork, I'll get either the knife, or the fork.

More prevalent; however, there is a big issue amid any form of discussion with respect to selling anything. The confusion is almost impossible to deal with. About four days ago, while we were traveling from home to Edmonton, I mentioned we should sell the acreage because it's becoming too much work, and I can't keep up to the maintenance. The conversation went into places I never want to tread. It took from our place, to almost Edmonton (approximately one hour), to calm her down, and get her to stop crying.

The first thing she did, is blame me for going behind her back, making secret arrangements with someone, pressuring her into making a deal, and even closing the deal without her. I try to rationalize with her that no deals have been made with anyone, and I'm not trying to pressure her; we are just discussing things between ourselves, and no one else! For some reason or another, she pictures someone that I can't relate to, and brings them into the conversation; someone she might have seen a week ago in a restaurant or somewhere else.

She will then switch to finances, and that never goes well. There seems to be no thoughts of reality regarding the selling process. She feels we are giving the house away, will lose all the money, and fears for what we will do next. Conversely, she likes to look at properties, and I feel that in her mind, she thinks we would buy one and simply move into it; she doesn't understand that we must sell our place first.

About a week later I mentioned selling our Volkswagen Westphalia Camper Van, and we basically went through the same process again (I'll never learn). This time I tried to rationalize that we could make money on the deal (no concept), then explained why the 'Westy' wasn't suitable for us, because it doesn't have a bathroom; she then got angry claiming I was saying it was her fault, and I was blaming her. Didn't take as long to calm her down; nevertheless, it is an uphill battle.

These are some of the issues I deal with; however, what you don't see is us having fun together. Yesterday we were going to Edmonton, and she was pointing at things and generally jabbering in a good mood for a good 15 minute. Couldn't understand a thing she was saying; however, she was happy. I usually dance around these misunderstandings, and let her enjoy her conversing. I encourage her to talk, and keep talking, no matter what she is saying.

We do laugh a lot, and fall into spontaneous singing in the car…something she was always too self-conscious to do before her affliction. There are many, many, many times we hug, and show each other appreciation for holding together through this minor issue of Alzheimer's. I know it's not a minor issue; regardless, I am so pleased to be able to be with her, and treasure every smile and triumph we share. Alzheimer's is not a problem when we can experience the good things. She is aware of what is happening, and says she's thankful I am supportive, and being with her. It's a mutual feeling, even though I know things will change. I'm living in the moment, and trying not to think of the future.

Regarding her health, I think the last Thyroid treatment is finally working. Beth is starting to gain a little weight, and that is good.

She likes to sleep a lot, which is great. We generally go to bed at 10:30 p.m. and she generally sleeps till 9:30 a.m., or sometimes, she will sleep in till 11:00 in the morning. When we do have to get up at 8:00 a.m., to go see dad, she does fine all day long.

Well, basically, that's what's going on with my precious. For me, I'm doing great, really! I don't have any depression at all, things just slide on by. I'm getting the sleeping pills under control, and can plan the dosage I need for the next day. The real blessing is that I haven't dosed off while driving since I started the sleeping pills. Before, I would dose off between home and Red Deer (35 Kms), and back; now I'm able to concentrate on driving, and enjoying the scenery with no drowsiness to speak of. The liquorish I bought to keep awake (if I'm chewing, I'm not sleeping) is now stale and hard. I do hit a fatigue stage during the day, usually once I'm back at home, and I get a half hour snooze before making supper.

I hope this helps explain what is happening, and at this time, everything is going as good as can be expected.

13 OCT, 2015

Happy twirty-sixth Anniversary to us, and I'm in tears! It's 8:16 a.m., and Beth is still sleeping, so I thought I'd take this opportunity to do a significant update, just to show you how fast things can change from three weeks ago

Beth is now to the point of almost incomplete comprehension, and now, her dreams are becoming her reality. We were visiting our son and daughter-in-law for Thanksgiving, and yesterday morning, when I woke up, Beth was almost completely dressed, worried about someone trying to sell our clothes. Had to get up as well, even though I needed more sleep. To add to the problem, my back was so sore I couldn't bend enough to put my socks on. The rest of yesterday didn't fare much better with more confusion and anxiety; there seems little to be thankful for, other than close family, good food, and Beth still with me…for now.

She keeps adding people to our space, there is always another person riding in the car with us. She talks about the two kids we were just with (usually two), even though our grandkids are sixteen and twenty-three, and we haven't seen any children for some time. She also sees little dogs along the road, usually a day or two after even seeing a little dog. She sees many things along the road that just aren't there.

One of the biggest issues I am facing, while we are traveling, is her voice drops to inaudible mutterings that I can't hear due to the wind, the road noise, and the tinnitus ringing in my ears. Additionally, I struggle to understand what she is saying, and can't.

Last night it became quite evident we must be careful as to what we watch on TV. That, in of itself, is also being added to her reality; just a documentary we watched that now is a major concern.

Of course, her reasoning is also being affected. I set things out for supper (utensils), and she will start to put them away before supper is finished cooking. Explaining to her we haven't eaten yet is not understood. It's best to just let her do her thing.

14 OCT, 2015

Quick update. Had a wonderful Anniversary yesterday, despite what I wrote in yesterday's update. Stayed focused on what Beth was saying, and wanted, and it worked out perfectly.

9 NOV, 2015

My second last post was written under duress, and perhaps sounded a little hopeless. Things haven't been that bad since, though they are deteriorating

I find she often substitutes words in a sentence. Something like 'nice day for a ride in the sink'; most times I can catch on to what she means. I sense she knows she didn't use the right word, and it frustrates her. I encourage her to keep talking because the last thing I want her to do is 'clam-up'.

She is now hearing things as she sometimes hushes me, and listens intently. She even says someone's talking. This happens in the car, so I know there's no one else with us. She often questions what I said, and once she repeats what she heard, I realize she can't hear me properly, as such, I must en-un-see-eyt (enunciate) my words more carefully.

Referring to my second last post again, I've determined the other person with us is some guy named 'Art' (me). While we were in the kitchen, she turned to the Living room, and asked Art what he thought. I'm not trying to make fun of the situation, as I understand what she is going through. Gratefully, I'm still a part of her life; however, at times the 'me' in front of her, is not the 'me' she recognizes. Perhaps, for her we have just been married, and I'm just some old fart she cooks with. I just thought it was cute, and I don't want to forget the good things that make me smile. Love her so much!!

A friend text me to suggested we get together, with another friend of ours, to celebrate his (14th Dec) and my BDay together. I read it to Beth, and she liked the idea; however, got upset that we weren't waiting for them when we left for breakfast. She couldn't understand that we were scheduling for a time a month away.

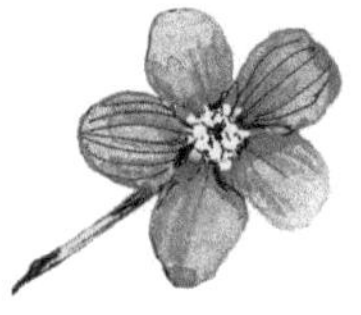

Chapter: Year 6

JAN 17, 2016

I feel we're entering a new phase of incomprehension, which has now regressed to about the three to four-year-old stage. Of course, she transitions upward on good days (or moments), it seems to depend on what we're talking about. I now feel the new stage in her care, is 'reasoning'.

Last night we stayed up till 11:30 p.m. (big mistake), and I could not get her to reason that it was bedtime. She didn't like her PJ bottoms, and eventually ended up in her jeans. At 12:30 a.m., she had shoes and a parka on, and I was afraid she was going to go outside at -20 below. We had a few words of discussion; however, she could not reason what bedtime was. I couldn't figure out where she was coming from, and nothing I said was understood. In retrospect, maybe she was just cold.

The latter has been happening a lot lately. She figures she's old enough to make her own decisions, and insists on doing so. Wish I could figure out what she wants to do.

FEB 12, 2016

Yet another phase is being entered. Both of us had the Flu which was a nightmare. My inability to speak due to Laryngitis, made her think I was yelling and spitting at her. Her vocalization, and comprehension, are down considerably, and I barely understand what she is trying to say. She sees people everywhere, regardless of if they are there or not, and talks to them constantly. The chairs have a better conversation than I am getting.

Most disturbing, is that her dreams are now reality, and at this juncture, patience on my part is tantamount. She will talk in earnest during the day about things she dreamt of.

At 3:30 this morning, I awoke to her trying to open the front door to let the boys (grandsons) in. She got really upset that "I didn't believe her", "I could at least go along with her". I hadn't confronted her, just asked why she was opening the door. I even opened the door to show her no one was there; regardless, the damage had been done. Kept calm, and she eventually settled down.

It's so hard to know how to handle such a situation. I could have just said nothing, or done nothing, and just wait for a queue as to what is acceptable as a next step for her. Alternately, I could have said "they must be late, and we'll just have to wait.", or the obvious, would have been to cause a diversion like saying, "Ok, let's just make a cup of tea, and wait for them." All of these would have been a better solution; however, at 3:30 in the morning, the mind is not always as quick as the reaction

As previously stated, I must reiterate that I must keep a very close eye on her now. Yesterday, she went to the washroom at Timmie's, I was sitting at the table keeping an eye on her and when she came out, she had no idea where I was… I had to get her, and bring her to our table. I feel that from this point on, I will have to stand guard at the door of the facilities.

Standing guard became the norm! If a lady was heading in to use the washroom, I would explain that my wife had Alzheimer's, and was using the facilities. It is amazing how understanding people are in this regard, and how many say they used to work in a care facility. Many times, I had to enter the lady's washroom to flush the toilet, and make sure everything was clean, something that became more and more common. At times I would have to attend Beth in a Public Washroom, if a lady would enter while I was in a stall with Beth, I would advise that I was in the stall with my wife; the response was always that of understanding. Eventually, I started using the men's washroom with her, and she was none the wiser.

Something to keep in mind, is that as things start to progress with this situation it is a good idea to start to remember which locations have a family washroom, and start to frequent those establishments. Such a blessing!

On an unrelated subject, she always follows, and doesn't want to lead, probably because she doesn't know which way to go. Being behind me makes it hard to keep my eyes on her, and of course, she hates it when I guide her in a direction. When leaving Timmie's, I went towards the door, and unbeknownst to me, she wandered the other way, sat down, and started to talk with a young couple. They were quite accepting, and didn't seem to mind the intrusion; perhaps they suspected, or recognized, that Beth had a form of Dementia.

It's hard to see her life, and personality, being stripped away, one layer at a time, like the leaves on a cabbage (there are not nearly enough layers on an onion).

28 FEB, 2016

How far removed do you have to be to have no negative responses, or emotions? I don't mean good emotions, like love, I mean those like being angered, agitated, self-righteous, anal, correct, whatever! When will I be so removed, that nothing she does will surprise me, and cause me to react negatively? Sometimes I get off on a tangent, get her upset, yet I stand my ground. This is not a good idea, I must re-evaluate my actions, and let her do what she feels she needs to do.

I can't emphasize enough how, for her, what she perceives as what she must do is a need, not a desire.

There are emotional responses in every relationship, it's all part of being a union. You have your views, you stick to them, you prove your point, you get upset, you argue, you go to bed angry, you wake up, you apologize, you make up, and life goes on. In an Alzheimer's relationship, the '***you***' mentioned above, must be nonexistent. You can never stand your ground; she is not capable of understanding your reasoning.

Last night we had Cranberry Chicken, Beth poked a hole in the tin foil, and the juices escaped, to which I responded with, "Why did you do that?" What she had done was not a big deal, and though not in anger, my response was inappropriate.

Later that evening she wanted two Tylenols, half an hour after she had taken two previously. I tried to convince her she couldn't take them because it was too soon, and that would be too many. After briefly arguing, I just walked away. That was wrong thing to do, as she was visibly upset; again, inappropriate of me. She probably had a headache, what detrimental effect would a couple more Tylenols have on her health. Another thing to note, is she doesn't forget that easily. When I apologized in the morning, she was in tears… so was I. I desperately must change my reaction!!!

If I want her happiness to be of prime importance, which I do, I must remove every bit of negative emotion, or response from our interaction. If you think it's easy, try it! I must be able to think first of how big an issue it is, consider the safety concerns, the consequences, determine how I can help her do what she wants to do, and then, how can it be fixed; all before I say or do anything! I call it, 'face the Tango of Reaction, or the Agony of Retribution!'

11 MARCH, 2016

I must report that following recommendations from my previous post, regarding removing emotion and reaction, are working. Very pleased, and in relation to the above, I'm discovering some basic laws to follow with respect to caregiving.

1. Always follow up on a hint. If she changes her mind, and wants to go somewhere else, it's for a reason.
2. You can't "teach her a lesson"! (i.e., If I let her have her way, and she fails, she'll learn). I don't mean this in a mean, derogatory, or dangerous way. What I'm referring to, is in relation to things that annoy me. First and foremost, she has no concept that what she is doing is out of the

ordinary, and she won't look at it as a lesson learned. Unless it poses a danger, let her carry on as normal, and fix it later.

3. Never make important changes, or decisions, because you assume "she won't understand anyway"! Her necessity to be involved, as in the past, has not changed. She understands inclusion is an important part of life, and though she may not understand, or be able to follow the process, she knows she should be involved to help decide on an issue. This is a hard one, some decisions must be made, and getting her positive involvement is crucial. Good Luck! What seems to work is proposing why the action must be taken with the 'Pros' positive to her as simple common sense (to her), and 'Cons' of what needs to be done. "Wouldn't it be nice to put a coat on, and be nice and warm, rather than getting cold with a chill?" Her agreement goes miles towards her wellbeing. And don't forget, you'll have to rehash this process many times over.

17 MARCH, 2016

The world is unfolding as is expected. Some people travel the world, and see the beautiful sights. My purpose is to take care of the love of my life. I feel privileged that I have been chosen for this purpose. I get to experience something that few people will ever do. It has strengthened our love for each other, and I have been transformed into a much better man, I hope!

Am I sad? Yes! Do I cry? Of course! Do I get frustrated? Absolutely! Do I get mad at Beth? How could I? Unfortunately, sometimes I do, then quickly reiterate to myself that it's not her fault; just another of '***MY***' issues, that '***I***' must overcome!! Do I blame God? Not at all! I thank him for the privilege of being chosen to take care of one of his special people. He must love her very much to have chosen me as that one, in that I will not give up on her.

Am I going to miss her when she's gone? Undoubtedly!! Nevertheless, only till I die!! So much so, that I will have no real reason to live on. My purpose in life will have been fulfilled; nonetheless, I'm sure the Lord has another purpose in mind for me. Maybe I'll become Prime Minister, maybe I'll solve the climate change issue, maybe I'll travel the world, and see beautiful sights, or maybe, I'll just join the Karaoke circuit. Who knows?

23 MARCH, 2016

A somber day indeed. Today was the day we implemented the Enduring Power of Attorney and the Personal Directive for Beth. Needless to say, I'm sad, and scared as hell! Her care is now fully my responsibility, and making decisions on her behalf will be necessary, and at times, very difficult.

10 APRIL, 2016

RestoraLAX Incident

Something for you to watch out for! We're at a stage where I must attend to Beth on bathroom breaks, whether at home or not. Beth was visiting the washroom for a bowel movement, and had very much difficulty in relieving herself; she was in a lot of pain. When she finally let go, the stool was very large, and hard. So much so, that it was too big for the drain, and could not be flushed down; I had to break it up.

This occurred again a week later, and I had to take her to Emergency, because she was 'Impacted', and unable to relieve herself. She was given an enema to ease the process which didn't help much. I was then advised to put Beth on a regiment of RestoraLAX, a stool softener. Things went well, yet after three or four weeks, I got lax on the treatment, and she got Impacted again. After this point in time, Beth was on a constant daily regime of RestoraLAX.

24 APRIL, 2016

It is Beth's Birthday, and I reflect on the love we've shared in the past, and the love for her that now overwhelms me. As such, I'd like to do a little monologue on my perception of 'Love'. Now, with this current birthday of Beth's, I ponder how much time I have left to love her, care for her, and most distressingly, be with her.

Love is an elusive, and illusive beast; nevertheless, what is it? Many have asked that question, and many have tried to answer, and yet, we still ask.

Love is a dedicated friendship; call it friendship or call it a union, love is the mitigating factor. You can love a person, and you can love everyone. You can love their facial features, their body. You can love the way a person makes you feel (happy), you can love the way they treat you, admire you, pamper you. You can love their mind (intelligence), their personality, the way they speak, laugh, smile. And don't forget the intimacy, etc., etc., etc.!!! In most cases, it's one, or a combination of some of the above, and yet, all these things are superficial.

Any of these things can change, and usually do, most often, not for the best. What happens then? Do you grow apart? Do you suffer through the changes? Do you remember how they were, and continue to live in the past? Do you stop loving them? In many cases yes, and in many cases, your love turns into intolerance, or hate. You will have arguments, fights, differences of opinion (and of course you are always correct). In most cases you patch things up, in some cases, you separate, and let go.

Love for oneself is tantamount to success in life. Without it, you have no purpose, no self-esteem, and no self-respect. All these factors are required to find true love with others. You must deal with whatever issues you have with yourself, and overcome them. NOTHING you perceive as a reason to dislike yourself is that relevant anyways.

Rejoice in the love others have for you, relish the things you bring to the table. Your dealings with, and the pleasure you bring to others, is an important part of their lives. You matter to a lot of people. If it's simply esthetics you are concerned about, look around you, and you will see your concerns are unfounded. There's always someone with more missing limbs, more mental issues, more sickness, and definitely, a worst hairdo!! Love yourself for what you are, don't hate yourself for not being what you want to be, or think you should be!

You must love yourself before you can love someone else, yet love for yourself can be a double-edged sword. Trouble is, some people love only themselves, everyone else is a trophy, bragging rights. Without tolerance, patience, and selflessness, there can be no love.

What binds some people together through all the changes? Some will continue to love the other person through thick and thin for some unknown reason… it goes beyond traditional wedding vows, "for better, for worse, for richer, for poorer, in sickness, and in health, and not until death do you part"!

Love! Still undefined; nonetheless, that is love!

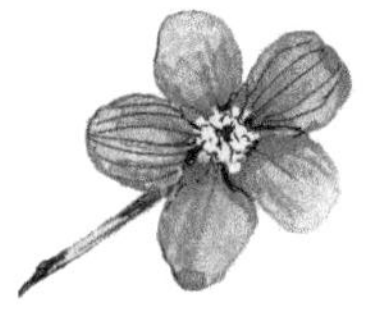

Chapter: The Necessity of Change

15 MAY, 2016

Lots has happened, and changes are coming quickly. We moved from Rimbey to Westlock, to be closer to family. This is where thinking of your finances also come into play. We had to sell our acreage, as I could not keep up with the maintenance and taking care of Beth at the same time, which in of itself, became overwhelming. It was, of course, a no brainer; problem being, it hadn't occurred to me that we would have to move at all; It bites, and I know I got screwed royally by the real-estate agent.

Last fall, we had a bank assessment on the house to refinance the mortgage, and the assessment came in at $370K. With all the work I did, in and around the house, I figured the acreage should have been worth around $425K; I had a twenty-eight foot by twenty-eight-foot heated garage, with a ten-foot ceiling, completely insulated, plywood walls, and ceiling, wired for 120V and 240V suitable for welding, and all the high powered, woodworking tools, you could imagine; most of which I owned.

In the house, I built a new, built-in wood burning fireplace, which cost me upward of $6K, and a brand new, completely gutted and finished bathroom on the main floor, complete with in floor heating, costing us over

$20K, just to start with. None of this was considered value added, as the bank deemed it to be standard fixings. Fair enough; however, before we listed, the agent said he wouldn't list the place for more than $305K; held my ground, and listed for $350K.

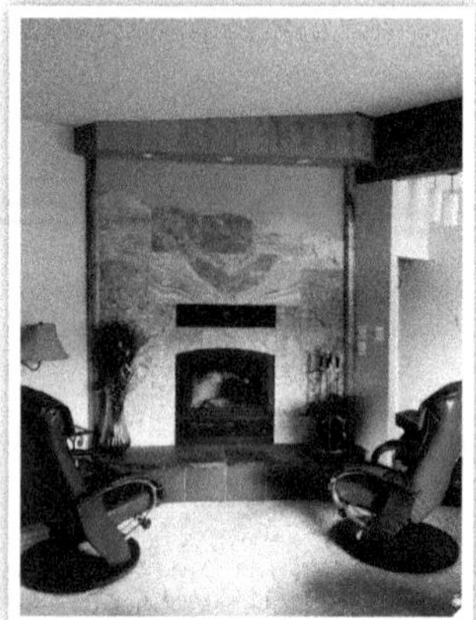

First bid that came in was for $305K, from a real-estate agent from Calgary… surprise, surprise!!!

This is where you hopefully have enough time on your hands to prepare for what must be done. I figure I lost at least $70K on the deal, nonetheless, being in a predicament, I took the offer… next day, an offer came in for $330K. Think ahead for what will have to be done, and save yourself a lot of money!! I lost a lot of money selling our private campsite location for the same reason.

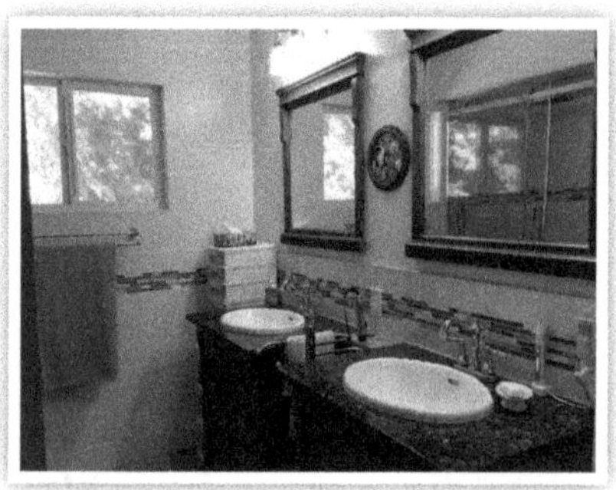

Regardless, we collectively enjoyed discovering our new surroundings, and the new places to eat. People here seem very welcoming, and understanding with respect to our situation. Beth adapted very quickly to the new Condo, the transition was seamless.

It comes to mind, that spouse caregivers will always run into a situation where, getting rid of stuff is always an issue. Even a piece of useless paper can be important to the patient! Best way I can understand this, is that these things reside in their current world. That's what they are familiar with and very important to them. In a disordered mind of an Alzheimer's patient, they must hang on to everything, for fear of having their whole world thrown upside down.

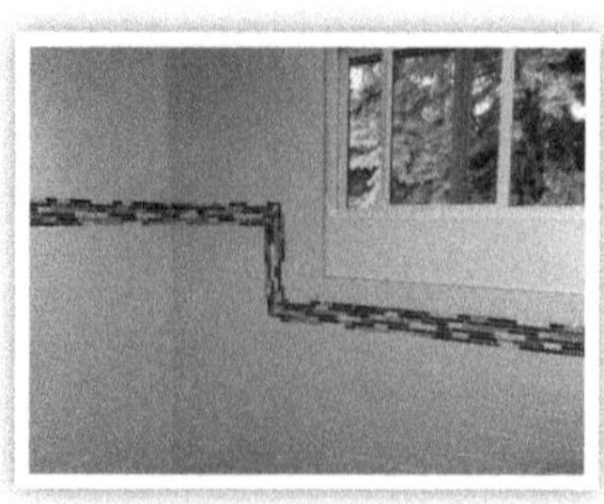

To determine what you are dealing with, if you need to downsize for a move, try removing something they don't use, though always in their space. I'm not referring to the living room suite, more so a picture, or a lamp. Don't throw it away in case it really means something to her, just hide it where she won't see it. If that works, proceed to remove other things slowly without her knowing.

The reason I mentioned the above is because that was the case with Beth. I had issues with downsizing, and packing things; however, once the move was completed, I was totally surprised that she didn't need, or even miss anything. It was a new world to her, and she was OK with it. Of course, I don't recommend changing anything significant, we still have the dining room suite, couch, bedroom furniture, etc., things she was familiar with.

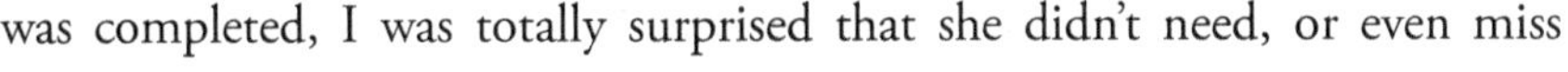

7 AUG, 2016

I started getting home care in to help Beth change into her PJs at night, and that seems to be working out well. I am also attending the local Alzheimer's Support Group once a month. It's interesting, that most of the people in attendance, are new to the game, and I find myself passing on my years of experience. It is a worthwhile endeavour for anyone experiencing this trauma in their lives. It provides a two-hour break for me, and gives the kids a chance to be with Beth to help them understand what I'm going through.

SEPT 2016

A month ago, I was goaded into getting someone in to provide me with respite of sorts. My first train of thought, was that I was alone a long time before I met Beth, and I will be alone a long time after she passes… why would I want to be alone now?? As I'm starting to climatize to the idea, it does give me a chance to either, get something done, or at least have an uneventful lunch at a Chinese Smorg.

Contrary to uneventful lunches, eating with Beth is becoming an issue. Going to a restaurant has been next to impossible lately. Beth will not sit down at the table, and/or she will take a few bites, then get up, and start to wander around.

One trick I learned, is to always request a booth, and have her sit in first, then sit beside her. It was hard to do at first, as we always would sit across from each other. Eventually, she became accustomed to this arrangement. Something you may want to start earlier in the process.

She is also this active at home, very hard to get her to sit at the table. I must guide her into the chair, and at times, reassure her the chair is there, "It's OK honey, the seat is behind you." She won't stay sitting at the table if there's no food in front of her. Food must be cut for her, as she can't use a knife to cut the food. To start her eating, the first bite must be offered to her on a spoon or a fork. Then, she will get up from table, and leave after a few bites, sometimes to look for Kleenex, a napkin, or water. She will then sometimes return, and eat more, sometimes not. At least at home, I can take my time till she finishes eating, though there is never enough time.

OCTOBER, 2016

Perhaps now is a good time to review Beth's daily routine for the sake of posterity, and for you to get a semblance of what your life will be like. This is what I consider to be an Alzheimer's, mid-late-stage assessment, for Beth and me, five years into the ailment.

Daytime will start about 9:30 a.m. She will go to the bathroom, take her meds, have breakfast, and usually go back to bed.

Gets up around 11:00 a.m., change from her PJs, and into her street clothes. Sometimes she goes back to bed.

Get up about 12:00 noon to eat lunch. Usually a sandwich.

After lunch, we either go for a drive, go shopping, or sometimes she goes back to bed.

3:00 p.m., usually go for Muffin and Coffee at Timmie's.

Prepare her RestoraLAX when we return.

6:00 p.m., start cooking. Eat about 7:00 p.m.

8:15 - 8:30 p.m., Home Care comes in to change her back into PJs.

Have a snack of Peaches, Yogurt, Chocolate, or Cheese.

Goes to bed between 9:30 p.m. and 10:30 p.m.

Will sleep until 12:30 a.m. to 2:30 a.m., go to Bathroom, and either go back to bed, or if antsy, ask if she's hungry, and she will say yes if so. Will then get a toasted peanut butter and banana sandwich, or toasted raisin toast with either honey and cinnamon, or jam.

Get up again at 5:30 a.m., or so, to go to bathroom. Often gets morning meds.

Go back to bed.

IDIOSYNCRASIES

Personality:

This is sad!! She no longer has any of the traits I fell in love with… the person she was. Her face always smiling, is now almost totally devoid of any emotion, except the occasional anxiety, and aggression. Sometimes there are fleeting moments of joy, as short as they are. There is no verbal interaction that you can understand; no responses that were always witty funny, or even serious. No joking around, teasing, or threats of retribution. NOTHING!!!

Medication:

She will sometimes take medicine by hand, or in a spoon. She won't be fooled by putting hard pills in pudding or other food. Sometimes she will spit the medication back into the water, and sometimes on the floor. Crushing, and mixing with food works best.

Sleeping:

Beth will sleep a lot, and has a tendency to sleep across the bed. She will often grab the sheets, and cuddle up with them on the bed. She will often get out of bed, and take all the sheets with her. Sometimes it's an issue getting her clothes changed in the morning and at night; nevertheless, with patience I manage.

Bathroom:
This is always a situation you never look forward to, and yet, must suck it up for! Bathroom is scary at best! She has problems getting her jean button undone. One issue you will run into is sitting properly on the toilet. At this stage I must attend to these necessities.

Learning:
She now seems to be at a two-year-old level; always on the move, and unaware of what she has unlearned. When kids are two years old, they are always learning things. As a parent the teaching process is special, treasured, and rewarding. Sadly, for a patient at this level, all you can do is watch them unlearn all they've ever known in their existence. You can't teach them the old stuff! So sad!

At this stage, I'm in a state of depression, and stressed with this nuance.

The Grip:
Beware the "Grip"! Beth tends to grab anything that passes in front of her, and hang on. She may be a whisper of a thing, although when she has a hold, watch out Schwarzenegger!

The reason I mention this, is that will be the most frustrating thing you'll have to put up with. Anytime you try to change her, she will grab on to a piece of clothing, and will not let go; undressing her for a change of clothes is a particular challenge.

Of course, I can overpower her, or at least try to, and sometimes I do; nonetheless, I must be careful not to hurt her. She will use words and tears I'm not accustomed to, with time, and patience; however, I do prevail. Sometimes it's best to just walk away for a few minutes, depending on what stage of disrobing she's at. Thing to remember is that she is oblivious to the fact she is holding on. It's not her fault, and specifically not her problem, it's mine!!

There are ways to get her to let go, best is to provide a diversion, and yet, even that sometimes doesn't work. You can try to suggest a reason to let go, such as, "Can I throw this in the wash for you?", "I just need to borrow this for a moment.", "You can get it back right-a-way.", sometimes just saying the words, "Can I have it please?", or even just, "release please". Each time is different.

Hyperactivity:

She tends to be hyperactive when she's awake. She likes to move things around, and picks everything off the floor. As she is wandering, she will at times wander towards the outside door. Not the time to take a nap!!

Yours is now a life of reaction, experimentation, and disappointment!

5 DEC, 2016

As of the beginning of December, Beth has started becoming more and more aggressive both towards the home care nurses, and me.

For myself, I'm finding that meaningful conversation is lacking, as is interacting with the community. We spend most of our time sitting on the couch, and listening to music with our photos as a screensaver on the TV. It certainly calms Beth, and I get a lot of rest.

23 DEC, 2016

Beth is regressing quite a bit daily. She is at a stage where the confusion and frustration are causing anger. I fully understand, and won't let it bother me. I'm starting to have problems getting her to eat, and take her medication. I don't know how long I will be able to keep her at home with me, and will base the decision on her health and wellbeing.

Of course, I love her very much, yet it is hard to be with your soulmate, and not be able to have even a small conversation. I guess that's one of the things I miss the most. Please don't feel sad for us though. As I've said previously, I feel I have been blessed, to have been chosen by the Almighty, to be the one to take care of such a special person.

24 DEC, 2016

Had Christmas dinner at my sister's place; a yearly family event always looked forward to and treasured. This year it was very noticeable to everyone that Beth was not the person we once knew. Not the kind of Christmas I was looking for.

Her captivating smile, her pleasant and cherished demeanour were no longer present. The expression devoid of any emotion, and the look of a total loss was disturbing to me. There was no laughter, there was no conversation to speak of; only direct responses that were not understood.

This Christmas there was no joy to share with the person I most enjoy being with.

31 DEC, 2016

No, this is not about wishing everyone a 'Happy and Prosperous New Year'.

She's so cute!! At 1:15 a.m., I was lying in bed when I woke to Beth rummaging in the bedroom; not a blanket or comforter to be seen!! How did she uncover me without me knowing?? Anyways, I looked all through the house until a closer look found the missing bed covers in the bathtub. So, I proceeded to recover the bed (while she was in it). I then sat, and fell asleep on the couch, only to be awakened at 2:15 a.m. by a quiet little voice of desperation coming from the bedroom saying, "Art". Upon entering the bedroom, I find the bed covers all twisted up in a pile on top of the bed, and her trapped inside. What exciting configuration of the bed sheets will I find in an hour??? Time will only tell.

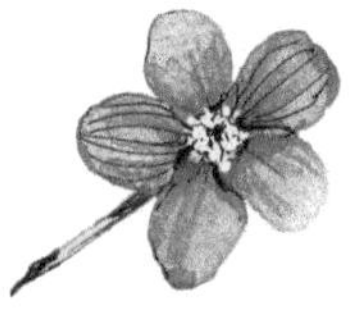

Chapter: Year 7

1 JAN, 2017

8:00 a.m. this morning I heard a bit of sound from the bedroom. Beth had gotten up, and walked straight into the closet. She was standing there clutching onto the cloths hanging up as though she was on the edge of a cliff, hugging the edge of the precipice. I talked her down, so to speak, and led her to the washroom. All the while she was in a state of mind resembling a trance. When I got her back to bed, she laid down in her current side fetal pose.

I realized she has been lying that way a lot in the last month or so. Not very observant, am I? I think it's a sign of the last phase of Alzheimer's; one in which she is close to the end of her ordeal.

It doesn't mean it's over, not by a long shot! Just that it signifies the beginning of the end of her consciousness. A sign that yesterday, I made the correct decision to start the placement process. It will be a long year. May God forgive me for putting such a dear person out of my circle of protection and care. The love and caring will still be there, yet I'll be on the sidelines.

This new reality will impact your psyche; placement is not an easy process. First thing to consider, is that government rules and guidelines make things as difficult for you as possible; not their fault, just the way it works. One of the factors you will have to deal with, is that when you first consider placement, you will be advised that there is a waiting list; secondly, you can never be told where on the waiting list she is! Actually, you might be told; it is nevertheless irrelevant, even if she is at the top, someone might jump the queue in front of your spouse due to prioritization, and the seriousness of the queue jumper.

Second problem is that there is no way of knowing how long she will be on the waiting list, especially if you want her to be placed in a desirable location… preferably close to home. There are usually options; nonetheless, the only available one might be hours away as I experienced when Beth required placement.

The third consideration is, and this is a big one; if a place becomes available for your spouse, yet you feel you are not in dire straits, and would like to keep her at home, you will only have one more shot before she goes to the back of the queue. It's a do or die situation! This is when you will be plagued with guilt regarding the decision you make for, or against, the placement. "Things are going well, am I just giving up??" "Will she hate me for moving her out of my care, her home?" "I'm doing ok with her care, what's the rush??"

You are faced with a dilemma, yet, the reality of your situation must preside! Again, caring for her is not so bad when things are going smoothly; however, things can change in an instance. Of course, you can force the situation if things get out of hand, and there is concern regarding her care or safety. They will make considerations regarding the seriousness of the situation; unfortunately, they can't just provide a room and a bed anywhere, at any time. If things become serious, she could be placed in a hospital, or at the first available location, and that might be at the other end of the province, or at least seem so. That's when you wish you would have placed her when a placement was offered, still, at the time she was doing good… AAARRRRGGGGHHHHH!!!

Digressing back to the Government issue, it behooves me to wonder why they can't look at the data, regarding how many placements are required this year compared to last year, and the year before, etc., then factor in how many have passed away this year, compared to last year, and the year before, etc., and then forecast that 'Next year we will need 342 new beds! Let's get on that…then increase the requirement by ten percent!!' Instead, we are faced with what's the situation? How serious is the situation? What's the priority? Which ones can wait? Are there places anywhere else in the world? All followed by, "OK Sir, we have a place for her, but you have to decide today!!!!!!!" It Stinks, it's stressful, and believe me; it is all too common!!!

10 JAN, 2017

Well, my worst fears were realized, bathroom issue while not at home. Had a hair appointment for her today, after we got to the hairdresser and took her coat off, she said she had to go to the bathroom. By now I use the men's room, and fortunately they usually have a large handicap stall.

Got to the bathroom in the mall a little too late, 'D' bomb!! Had to cut her undies off, and fight her to clean up. She was constantly holding her pants with no sign of releasing, trying to pull her jeans up while I was trying to wipe. It seemed like a battle, or even a potential sex crime, going on in the stall. Thank God no one walked in on us. Cancelled the haircut, went home, and had a shower. Beth's resting in bed now, all squeaky clean in her PJs.

Wanted to spare you the details; nevertheless, this is what you can expect if you love, and want to care for your loved one.

JAN 29, 2017

What do you do when you reach the realization that you are slowly losing the one you love? When you know you will never share the same kind of love you've had together? When you recognize the one you love in a picture, more than the person in front of you? When you're giving your heart and soul to the person in front of you, yet it's never enough! You love her more now, though in a different way. There are no more laughs together, no more conversations, no more sharing. Does she love you? Of course! Does she understand you love her, probably? Does she know who you are…

I forgot to take my antidepressants for a couple days, and I consciously decided to wean myself off them last night. I'm back on them tonight! I guess I'm not ready yet.

FEB 17, 2017

Reflection On Today's Reality!

At some point in my life, I figured we had it all. Toys, dirt bikes, three vehicles at once including a Jeep Rubicon, a fishing boat, two motorhomes, a cabin in a private campground with a ninety-nine-year lease, a timeshare on a ski hill, home on an acreage next to a lake. Most importantly, had sufficient pensions, and a supportive, intelligent, and loving spouse. Yes, we had arguments; however, the makeup was quick, and forgiving. You name it, been there done that!! We lived life to its fullest, and could not want for more. I figure maybe that's when God had to knock me down a peg.

In the last six years, my life has been totally transformed. Beth has contracted Cancer, Hyperactive Thyroid, Alzheimer's disease, and now has Shingles. Because of my wife's condition, I have had to cease any existence I once knew. Basically, no more socializing, recreation, or entertainment! That means quitting the Rimbey Lions Club, and Citizens on Patrol (COPS), no more recreational activities, no dining out, going to movies. It also means no more woodworking, nor any form of home renovations, and…I've pretty much become celibate

A life of excess has transformed into complete and utter devotion, and commitment to the care of Beth. I've had to start doing all the shopping, all the cooking, all the dishes (we have no dishwasher), all the laundry, all the cleaning, all the yard work, schedule all the appointments! Essentially, do everything that is to be done around the house et all.

After my own personal care, I must dress my wife, attend to her personal care, schedule her medication, assist her to eat, assist her to shower, assist her to sit down anywhere, assist her to walk, assist her to go to the bathroom, and then assist her sanitization afterwards. I must attend to my wife 24 hrs a day, 7 days a week.

Tomorrow is yet another 'ground hog day', and you do it all over again because this is your life! I'll struggle to get her to change clothes, to get her to sit for meals. I'll reintroduce myself to the scent of facilities requirements. I'll accomplish three meals, and a snack. I'll meet the challenge of washing the dishes, and making the bed. I will attempt to succeed in getting her to take her medication. I might even get a couple loads of laundry in… "Oh my God, I've dusted"!!

I can no longer understand what my spouse says nor, can I have any form of conversation with her. In fact, our lives consist of sleeping, eating, watching TV, and pooping! That's all we do together now; nonetheless, I have no regrets, and would not shrug my duties for a minute. It disturbs me that she is not the person she was, and yet I am truly grateful to have her with me.

I now realize what is most important in my life, and I accept the reality of what God has provided me. I've learnt the only thing you can count on in life is change, and hope you to have the insight to survive through it all.

This is a disease, not unlike any other except it is termina; sometime within the next twenty years! There is no hope of recovery, or remission. You lose your soulmate with diminishing dreams, goals, and accomplishments together. Those were the bonds that made life worthwhile, and kept you together. You now see your life waning, one smile at a time, one kiss at a time, one hug at a time, and one memory at a time. You had it all, and now the life you once lived is just a memory.

Regardless, none of the things that defined my life matter, nor do they have meaning anymore. Ultimately, all that matters is that I get to see who she becomes, for possibly the next fifteen years… then, remember whom she was. At times, I feel abandoned by all but my friends and family, of which I get to enjoy the company of far too little.

APRIL 7, 2017

Beth currently sleeps a lot; I'd estimate twenty hrs. a day! Except when she gets up on her own, to go to the bathroom, I must wake her to change her clothes, and eat. I took the chance to go shopping for food yesterday; I would only be gone for twenty minutes, and I was sure she would sleep through my absence. I was able to breath the fresh air, able to drive at my leisure, roll down the window, hear the traffic. In the grocery store I was free to push my cart where I wanted, looked at the different types of dishwashing soap, turn down an aisle I knew didn't have anything I needed.

I was able to converse with the teller, share a bit of wit… "I had exactly twelve items, I was worried I might get kick out to another line."; "Oh, I have to pay for this?"; "No, I'll save my points till I'm a millionaire!"; "Thanks to the five cent a bag charge, the cupboard next to my sink is worth $5,000!". It all flowed out, and it was very important for me to just be able to talk or joke around with someone. I smiled!! Now, I have to go home, feeling much better. I hope Beth slept through my absence… didn't move a muscle!!

And then comes Thursday! For the last two months, I have been provided with three hours of respite a week; increased to four hours, as of the beginning of February. You open the door, step out of the house, and you're eyes open to a new world, full of possibilities! Thoughts fill your head; your heart is filled with excitement.

That's when I realized the importance of respite! Oh, the freedom! My dad is ninety-four years old, and with the four hours afforded me, is just enough time to visit my dad at his care centre in Edmonton. It takes me an hour and a half to get there, which gives me one hour to enjoy lunch with him if I get there in time. If I'm late, he will have started lunch, and I shouldn't disturb him. Then, an hour and a half to get back home, and to Beth.

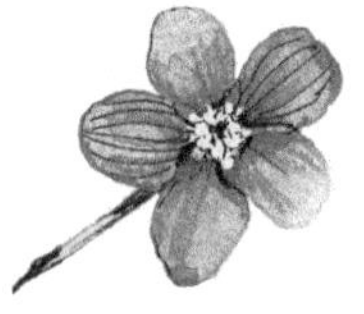

Chapter: Till Death Do Us Part!

15 MAY, 2017

That's it!! My back went out taking care of Beth, and man did it hurt! Called placement, to tell them I couldn't continue taking care of Beth on my own. You can't imagine the concept of telling someone your through…take them away!! It's a feeling of guilt you can never reconcile, and yet, you know there is no other option…you've done your best. So, you try to justify the fact that it is best for them, and yourself; nevertheless, failure comes to mind.

Got a call back from the Placement Office, and there was a misunderstanding regarding Beth's placement. There was a room available, if Beth was in the hospital. The room was booked for someone on the waiting list, and Beth could take precedence, but only if it was an emergency. Advised them that it wasn't an emergency for Beth, I was the one in dire straits. As it turned out, I wasn't expecting immediate placement, and after a consultation, Beth was not considered acceptable for this placement, and I would receive documentation to review other temporary placement options.

This is something I hadn't considered earlier on in the care process. As previously stated, it's a good idea to have the knowledge of the placement process in place, and be prepared before it's too late. It's a hard decision to make at the best of times, and worse under duress.

18 MAY, 2017

Received a Placement letter giving me a couple options for Placement. One, in the town we lived in, to which she was already on the placement list. Another was in a town 45 KMs away with yet another waiting list. The third, was 100 KMs away in which there were two Extendicare facilities. I was advised that there was a room available in one of the latter locations, and that if I chose it, once placed at a secondary choice location, she would be raised on the priority list for a move to the local care centre.

And then it hits you.

There comes a time when you can do no more. All your doing is upkeep. Memantine is a drug commonly used in the treatment of Diabetes Neuropathy that showed some promise with Alzheimer's patients, although only effective once the patient is in the latter stages of Alzheimer's. Apparently, Donepezil (Aricept) is not as effective anymore in leveling off the swings in brain activity levels that cause changes in mood, activity, and alertness… so they say. Well from what I see, they're wrong.

Beth was put on Memantine, and I was instructed to take Beth off Donepezil! After three days she regressed to not being able to eat by herself, and totally unable to walk on her own. She lies in bed in an almost comatose state. Her eyes slightly open when she looks at me except, she's not looking at me; she sees right through me. I want desperately to hold her and kiss her; however, all I can do is cry. That's the feeling of helplessness! That's when it hits you; I can't do this anymore… I need help!

By now it's Sunday of a long weekend, May 21st, and I haven't been able to contact her doctor. In desperation I tried to get a hold of the Hospital Emergency Ward, to see if I can put her back on Donepezil, and combine it with Memantine, I'm not versed on combining drugs. All they would say is to bring her to the Emergency ward. There is no way I can get her there on my own. In desperation, I called 811, and a Nurse suggested I call Poison Control. Great advice, I finally got someone, and they said the two drugs do not counteract each other, and there should be no problems combining the two. ***As a caveat: DO NOT DO THIS ON MY ADVICE!!! It might react to whatever else the person you are caring for is taking, or they might even have an allergic reaction!!!***

The result was swift, and amazing! With the combination of the two drugs, the next day she was back to her former state. After reviewing with the doctor, we decided to keep her on both drugs for the foreseeable future.

I swore I'd be her support till the end. I figured it would strengthen me, and make me tougher… a better man! Here I am blubbering in the corner, helpless! Love transcends the changes you face and see. Beth has changed from the bright, loving person I fell in love with, to a shell of a person she used to be. With the regressive changes she's gone through; I've just grown to love her more and more.

JUNE 3, 2017

Took a trip an hour away to check out the suggested Extendicare facilities. The furthest town is somewhere between here and nowhere. If it's not here, it must be there, and when you get there, you're nowhere. It's little more than a pitstop in the middle of the long road on the gateway to the North. Regardless, it is a nice, quaint little town, with friendly people bearing smiling faces. The town was once the centre of attention in Alberta, when four RCMP Officers gave up their lives in an ambush by a deranged person. Tragically, they left young families and friends behind to grieve for them. Needless to say, all of Alberta, and Canada grieved!

I arrived in this quaint little town, and looked for the Extendicare facility… it didn't take long. There are two care centres in town, one is a modern facility, attached to the Hospital. The one where Beth was to be placed was older yet quite nice. The kind of place I wouldn't mind residing in, what I envision as an old folk's retirement home.

5 JUNE, 2017

I've been contemplating life lately, after all I have seventy years of experience. At this age, it would be inherently silly to contemplate death, it's not that far away anyways! This is not the life I wanted; however, it's the life I swore to uphold!

Eventually, the crises are too much to bear, and you know it's time to let the professionals take over. Like a friend of mine said, "It's a hard thing to do despite knowing it's the best decision for all concerned. There are residual guilts, and tears, in odd places, there's even guilt about feeling relieved. The main thing; however, is knowing that your loved one is safe, and you can work on getting yourself help to better support them".

I contacted the Placement Office, and accepted the placement that was available! The decision is made, the process is started! Beth will be placed at that Extendicare facility tomorrow.

Got a VERY uplifting story to tell you about enacting this decision, you won't believe it!! Immediately after getting off the phone with the placement centre, I returned to the Livingroom love seat where Beth was sleeping. I had pictures on the TV from the shared Photo Album on my computer, and music playing from my iPhone through the Apple TV Box. That's when God spoke to me visually and musically, in correlation regarding my decision and action. Visually with the photo of three crows flying in a formation that depicts God smiling, and musically with a Randy Travis song called "Road to Surrender" saying, "My life is in your hands… help me let go of all the guilt that's held me under its control!" Coincidence? Yes!! Divine Providence? I think so; nonetheless, you decide!!!

This may be a good time for me to advise that you consider your finances.

It is so expensive to place Beth into a care facility, and as we saved for our retirement, there are no subsidies for us. Consider that just the care facility costs are a minimum of $2,000 a month, and that's for the cheapest government funded place in Albert. Some facilities can cost upwards of $5,000 a month. That means, the cheapest placement will cost a minimum of over $24,000 a year, on top of everyday expenses. Ask yourself if you can afford that right now?? I had to pay the full shot of Beth's care, and yes, I was able to claim it on my taxes; however, the tax claim refund was minimal.

Speak of the Devil, taxes will become an additional burden; what is claimable, what isn't? Then, when tax time comes around, and you reek the benefits of your unfortunate situation, the taxation arm of your lovely government will foster the belief that you are the lowest scum of the earth, and are cheating on your taxes. I went through five audits in the last four years of Beth's life, and the year following her death. When your life is at the pit of your existence, the last thing you need is to justify why you farted on a Friday!! Am I bitter… perhaps a bit!

It seems ironic that they are called 'Civil Servants' when there is nothing civil about them. I'm not looking for pity or revenge, I fully understand they are doing what they are supposed to do, and if I owe taxes, I'm more than willing to pay them; it's just the way they go about it. The first two audits resulted in me getting more back than I claimed.

The reason they audit you is simply because you are claiming more this year than last. Don't believe that they are randomly picking you from out of a crowd, as they claim; that's just an excuse to justify their unempathetic ways. They demand that you review every cent rather than analyzing why the refund was increased. If they would have done that, they could see that there is a reason.

Ok, off my high horse!! It's important to know that you must make sure you fill out your taxes correctly; actually, perfectly! I know of one lady that used an accounting firm to finalize the estate resulting from her husband's death. They submitted the wrong form in doing a transfer of the assets rather than an assimilation of the estate. They were married, and it should have been a 'no brainer' that she gets the house! The results were that the taxation department considered this to be a transfer of funds, and demanded that she pay $75K in back taxes; at one point they even sequestered her pension! Four years later, the tax department finally relented that, "OK, it was an inheritance, not a wage!" Sorry, I got back on the horse!!

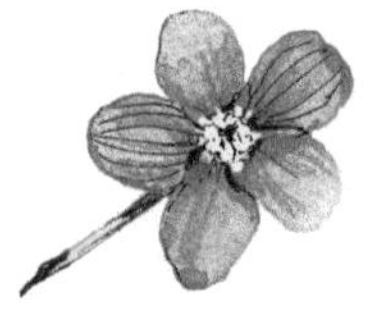

Chapter: The Separation

7 JUNE, 2017

Today Beth was admitted into the Extendicare facility 100 Kms from home. It went quite well; better than I expected actually. I am so fortunate that she doesn't equate this transition to being abandoned or losing her home, as many patients do.

This is where the Personal Directive comes into play for real. It may seem easy to make decisions at the time the Directive was made; however, when the time is at hand, there is considerable anxiety in enacting said Directive.

A Personal Directive outlines, and legalizes your wishes for level of care. A Power of Attorney empowers you to make that decision on behalf of the other person, and you must! If you've ever had to put down a beloved pet, you understand that of which I speak. The decision is the same, except the morality, and guilt, will be almost unsurmountable.

There will always be doubt as to whether you, and/or your spouse have made the right decision, especially, when you must enact that decision on behalf of your spouse. You will be put to task to render a decision, to a doctor, when an incident occurs. Worst case scenario is that it will become your decision as to whether they are to stick tubes down throats, and/or veins, or not; or even apply resuscitation efforts to keep your spouse alive when the prognosis is grim. The choice is never easily made, and not a decision you will want to make at the last moment without knowing your spouse's wishes.

Level of care will be discussed with administration upon placement. Her directive will be taken into consideration, and your decision will be administered should an event occur in your absence. Your decision does supersede, and take precedence, as a final decision in dire circumstances. It is confusing, and if you have any questions, seek advice from your lawyer.

Beth and I did not want to be resuscitated, and as an example, I will not be subject to chemotherapy should that be an option; it would be hard to make that decision on behalf of Beth. This must be discussed!!!

Once we got registered, we went to the dining room where they had a small band playing music. Beth was so enthralled, she got up, and started dancing on her own, dancing around the room by herself. The only reason I didn't get up and dance with her, is that I was taking a movie with my iPhone; something that I am so happy I did, something I get to treasure to the end of my miserable days.

One of the attendants started dancing with Beth, and she was in her glory. Beth then left the attendant, and started dancing across the floor on her own again. The floor was a Laminate style that looked like Barnwood Boards. Beth was dancing around, and suddenly, she started stomping on one spot. I figured that maybe she saw a spider… it was an imitation knothole, funny!!

She then gradually headed for the exit doors, still dancing, as if no one would notice. The doors are locked to prevent the residents from getting out, so I wasn't overly concerned, nonetheless, I figured 'oh, oh, here we go!!' Didn't work out that way at all, she just tried the door, then turned, and tried to pick something off the floor; happened to be an enclosed poison mouse trap… that got the attention of the attendants; it was all OK.

I would like to reinforce the importance of capturing videos of your loved one while you can… so precious… so treasured!!!!!!!

9 JUNE, 2017

Yesterday was one of the most sorrowful days of my life! I heard of the passing away of a dear friend of mine, after losing his brave three-year battle with Cancer. My dear friend, you will be missed; until we meet again in heaven! To the family, you have my sincerest condolences, my heart, and my prayers go out to you.

Yesterday my heart was aching, many tears flowed, and are still flowing for another reason as well. This deepened sorrow that befell me yesterday in this ongoing battle with Alzheimer's! That rotten disease has taken my wife away from me, in that I could no longer care for her properly. She was taken out of my care, and placed in an Extended Care Facility!

I in no way want to belittle the passing away of my dear friend, and I hope they forgive me; theirs was the greatest loss of all. The tragic loss of my friend supersedes my emotional loss of Beth under my care; however, the culmination of both losses within two days, combined with the realization that I too must also face the eventual loss of my loved one is almost too much to bear. Alzheimer's is a battle that no one wins!

17 JUNE, 2017

Not a good day for Beth, nor me. Beth is really disoriented today, and had a fall this morning. She seems to be ok; however, very sleepy. I guess this is what life boils down to, there is nothing in the world that I would rather do than sit here, beside Beth, as she sleeps.

It's an opposing emotion filled day, and it's hard to figure which emotion will win out; nonetheless, neither can. When you see your loved one in an almost comatose state, you want to do something; unfortunately, you can't; you're sad you can't do anything for her; however, you're happy that she's a place where they can provide better care; you're sad she's not home with you, yet, you're happy she's in a home; you wish she were the person she was, and yet, you see her as the person she is; sadly, you want her to get better, and again, you want her to pass away to be released of this curse. I guess it all boils down to the difference between your wishes, and her needs, and both are at the opposite ends of the scale.

The guilt you feel is that you were taking care of her 24 hrs a day, now can only stay with her for a few short hours. You wonder if, and wish you could do better, yet know you can't. Through it all, the tears flow!

22 JUNE, 2017

After Beth's fall, I contacted the Placement Coordinator, and within two days she was able to find a room in the Westlock Continuing Care Centre. This did come as quite a surprise; I was told to have Beth at the care centre TODAY!!!

Seems funny, I was ecstatic that Beth was moving close to home, and yet never in my life have I ever felt so useless, worthless, helpless! Combined with the loss of a dear friend, a couple weeks ago, I was feeling overly depressed in that there was nothing I could do to change things to make Beth better, yet I know it's not me, it's this damn Alzheimer's sucking the life out of me!!

That's how Alzheimer's effects the caregivers and loved ones. It's a curse, the rational of which I would like to transfer onto someone; however, no one holds responsibility. I can't blame God for Alzheimer's, or any other man-made diseases like Cancer or MS, or any other curse for that matter. God created the perfect world, man screwed it up.

Think of it, Alzheimer's must be a man-made, or simply a human condition, not something brought on by the powers that be, selecting you… or her… or them, for no specific rational whatsoever. There are mad and evil people all over the world, why would God take the best and kindest, and inflict them with any of these catastrophic and terminal diseases; is he lonely? We pray for remission in the hopes that God will answer and save, yet it never comes (well, mostly never).

No matter how bleak, or lost, or hopeless you feel, count the blessings in your life, there are many; the sunshine, the rain, the flowers, mostly; however, your friends and family… and God!!

Well, my friends, it didn't take long to get an answer from The Almighty, here's what happened!!

I was transferring Beth to the Extendicare facility in in our Village today. At about 10:00 a.m., I was driving along with Beth at my side when a squirrel ran in front of the car, and I had no opportunity whatsoever to dodge him.

In my vulnerable state, I felt a twinge of remorse, my only hope was that the little guy paused under the car, and went on his merry way. Unfortunately, a glance in the rear-view mirror revealed the outcome.

I know most of you wouldn't think twice of this situation; however, I had to wonder why? With an absence of trees for a quarter mile, and nothing except a small bush near the road, where in the world did he come from? With no trees around… why was he even there? Combine that, with two miles of straight road in front of me, one mile behind, and not a car in sight, why would this Squirrel wait for me to come along, and dash out at the most inopportune time? Coincidence? Perhaps suicidal?

The feelings of this morning reverberated with me. Again, I felt sorry, yet mostly helpless that I couldn't avoid the poor little guy. That's when it occurred to me that we must deal with these feelings of uselessness, hopelessness, and helplessness in facing the inevitable! Perhaps this squirrel was sent to show me that, as such, life in of itself exists only so we can learn, and feel emotions of all sorts. Life would be a pretty bland existence without such feelings.

Like I said most of you will figure I finally went over the deep end; nonetheless, if you can come up with even an inkling of why this happened, at the most inopportune time, at the most unlikely spot, for the most unlikely reason, I'll be more than happy to listen. I feel the good Lord talks to us all the time; all we have to do is sit back, and observe what's going on around us. As such, I believe he answered my remorse to let me know that these distressful feelings are ok and normal. Life happens; we must deal with it, and move on.

For the squirrel, he had to die as did my friend… for Beth, she has Alzheimer's, and there's nothing I can do or could have done about it. We're all going to die, we're all in the same boat, we're not unique, and thankfully we're not alone! Enjoy the journey while you can, observe and learn, love with all your heart, mostly though, expect to feel every emotion possible; still, don't let it ruin your life!

Perhaps I'll meet my little squirrel buddy in the great bye-and-bye, and thank him for the lesson. Maybe I can make it up to him, and we'll share a peanut together.

29 JUNE, 2017

Recorded another video of Beth dancing, I'm counting my lucky stars. In Westlock, they have the residents sit in a semi-circle, and either play kick the ball, or on this day, they played some music. Well, this was right up Beth's alley!! She got up, and started going up to the residents, all of which were wheelchair bound, and visited while dancing, sort of like we all do on the dance floor when we just face each other, and wiggle around in our enticing mating dance of attraction. She moved to different residents much to their pleasure. She went to one resident, and said, "I'm six years old!" It was funny at the time; however, I wonder if she might have actually believed that. The video is, again, priceless!!

13 AUGUST, 2017

Another sad milestone has been reached! Beth lost her balance, fell backwards, and had to have stitches to the back of her head. This is significant because it signifies her sense of balance is waning; she can no longer be trusted to walk on her own, and a wheelchair is now a major requirement for mobility; another consideration of your finances, especially the type that provide additional comfort in the ability to recline, they're not free.

Adding to the sadness is the fact that she does not know how to wheel the chair around on her own. I'm thankful I can be there to guide her around; such is not the case for a majority of the patients in this residence. The realization sets in that most of the patients here are dependent on the care attendants to move them from the bedroom to the table, to the TV set, where they then sit till the next meal; so sad!! That will not happen to Beth!!

Sightseeing trips have been reduced since her placement, and now I feel they will predominantly come to an end. Not that I can't take her, more so that she gets confused and agitated with all the movement and having to just sit there, potentially uncomfortable.

13 OCT, 2017

Happy 38th Anniversary, my love!!

This is a bitter-sweet day for me. There is nothing I **wouldn't** do to change the situation we are in, and there's nothing I **would** do to change our situation. I know it sounds oxymoronic, yet, let me explain.

It hurts me to see Beth as she is today. She is in quicksand, sinking slowly, and I am chained to a tree. I don't have an axe, or a saw, and there isn't even a Beaver in sight. There is nothing I wouldn't do to help her or change places with her in an instant! We all know what Alzheimer's is, and the results are inevitable. Essentially, there is no hope, and that is sad! Conversely, I wouldn't change one moment in my life since the first day I joined AGT, and fell in love with the personality and voice of the dispatcher that would eventually become my wife. I would marry her again in an instant, even knowing the outcome. I have been truly blessed to find my soulmate in this world, as many of my friends can attest.

Alzheimer's is a part of life many of us must deal with. It's no one's fault, it wasn't brought on by a curse of God, and the solace of knowing we will still be loved, and cared for by those we love, is the only thing we can hold on to.

Don't feel sorry for me as there is no place I would rather be or anyone I would rather be with than with Beth. I have been, and am, blessed! Don't feel sorry for Beth either, that's the last thing she would have wanted. Just be happy for both of us in that we are fulfilling our dreams of growing old together. One life too short, one not short enough; temporarily absented until we meet again. That's life!!

5 NOV, 2017

It's so nice to be old when you can rely on the wisdom of ages to prepare for all situations. We're doing a time change to transition back to Standard Time from Daylight Savings. This year, I thought ahead, and in preparation, I started to go to bed earlier, and to getting up earlier, to outsmart the system.

So, how did that work out for me?? Let me tell you!! Normally I go to bed at 10:30 p.m., and get up at 7:00 a.m., to do my morning constitutionals, so I can wake Beth up at 8:00 a.m. Now, I've been going to bed at 9:30 p.m., and getting up at 6:00 a.m. to prepare for Standard Time. This morning I woke up bright eyed and bushy tailed at…5:00 a.m.!! What the hell just happened?? It's supposed to be 7:00 a.m.!!!!! Now, I won't be able to keep my eyes open past 8:30 p.m.!! Damn!!

That's it! In the spring, I'm going to be smarter!! I'm going to go to bed later, and wake up later. They won't catch me this time!!

7 DEC, 2017 - THE DARK SIDE

As I experience my 71st Birthday… Happy Birthday to me!!… I contemplate my existence. The following thoughts are simply the wandering thoughts of a distressed mind; however, I thought them relevant enough for them to be revealed. Mine is but one experience out of millions, and I can't speak for anyone else; you might not feel as I do, as it might be unfathomable to have such thoughts. In this document I have stated that there are no holds barred. I haven't researched with anyone else so take It for what it's worth.

And now for the answer to the questions you don't want to ask. The Question? Do I ever desire that she would die, and I'd be free of this burden?

Actually, that's two questions. To answer the first, yes, I do. Not often, more as an occasionally fleeting thought. This is the woman I love, and am dedicating every effort possible to making her life as pleasant for her as possible. "In Sickness and in Health" was part of our wedding vows, and I'll be there for her till the end. Wishing she would die is harsh, and a misnomer; it relates more so to having to see her the way she is. It breaks my heart to see her in a constant state of fear, anxiety, confusion, and frustration. She's not the person I married, yet I still love her, and even more so now in her vulnerability. I morn for her every day. I must go through the five stages of grief all the time, many times over; and yet again, as I'm writing this book!! Shakespeare's words that "a coward dies a thousand times before his death" may be true; nevertheless, the brave can as well. I must be strong for her, it's not an option!!

Second part of the loaded question: I do think of what I will be able to do when she's gone. So many things come to mind. I think most prevalent, is to hit the road, and tour Canada and the USA… if a wall hasn't been built. It's probably unrealistic, and simply a form of escape; nonetheless, foremost in a disturbed mind. I guess the main question I need to consider is companionship. How do I just transition from loving, sharing, and caring, to me, me, me?? One thing that scares me the most is having to go through this again with another partner. I'm a caring person, that's been proven; nonetheless, I don't think I could live through this again!! I keep thinking a dog would be a good alternative, yet is that just another form of escape?? Would the escape last or just become a burden? What state of mind will I go through when I have to put it down?? I guess anyone's guess is as good as mine.

You know, this is a long, and emotional journey… very long; very emotional!! It provides you with a lot of time to think and ponder every potential aspect of this tumultuous disease. It all seems so hopeless right now, and a subject I referred to earlier comes to mind, 'Abandonment'! As I mentioned earlier, I would never consider this option; nevertheless, abandonment can be derived from the doubt and denial of the benefit you are providing to your partner, whether able to or not.

Some may think that it is pointless to be by her side constantly, because you are not able to help, or sometimes are not even recognized. I can assure you that throughout your lives together, she has depended on you for security and protection, and just because she has a temporary lapse of memory, doesn't mean she doesn't need that support; it is what she needs most now!!! Unfortunately, I see so many cases where a patient is visited once a week, or even once a month… some, not at all.

I realize that some people are not as fortunate as I, and must attend to the commitments and the requirements of their life. Fortunately, my situation is such that I can be with my wife every day throughout this disaster. In retrospect, if you love your spouse, the rewards, and peace of mind of attending to your spouse, as much as possible, will be worth it. The decision; however, is not an easy one, yet must be yours to make.

Just a thought, "Live Life to its Fullest!" is a misnomer! Properly translated it could mean "Live Life to its Shortest!". Living life to its fullest means doing everything possible, so as to experience everything life has to offer. It implies climbing the highest peak; breaking speed records on land, sea, and air; swimming the deepest ocean; sampling every drug known to man; all of which is detrimental to life! I profess it should read, "***Enjoy*** Life to its Fullest!!"

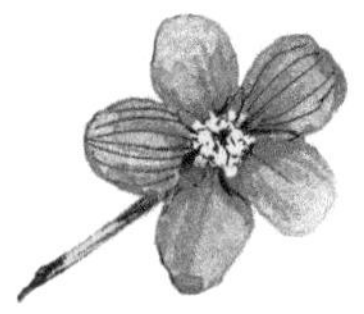

Chapter: Year 8

8 MAR, 2018

Had a wonderful moment today! Beth said, "I'm so Lucky!!" followed by "I Love You!" and stretched forward for a kiss!! This was done without prodding, just out of the blue… brought tears to my eyes!!! Makes every day in the past worth it, and gives me strength to look forward to everyday into the future! That's what love is!!!

As my sister responded, "Love always somehow transcends the impossible to touch your heart".

12 APRIL, 2018

My heart sang last night!! Dear friends of ours from Calgary dropped in for a visit, and there was Rum to be shared. A wonderful visit; however, what made my heart sing was the smile on Beth's face when we woke her from her sleep, and she saw her friend's face. The smile was instantaneous, genuine, and ear to ear! For an instant, Beth was back!!

Beth had many close friends, and this one was from way in her past. Beth was instrumental in getting these two wonderful souls together, and was bridesmaid at their wedding. To show how small the world really is, before we got married, and while sending out invitations, Beth mentioned her friend's name. I was familiar with the last name, as it is quite common; however, when she mentioned her husband's first name…

I'm not kidding!
As I'm writing this, I got an Alert on my Apple Watch,
iPhone, and Computer that Beth has to go for
Thyroid Bloodwork in 30 minutes.
It's now November 24th, 2020, and
as of today, Beth passed away
over 2 years ago. I had erased this alert
after her Thyroid issue was stabilized,
about 2 years prior, and I hadn't
received an alert since then.
This alert has magically set itself up again!!!

Hi, Beth! Miss you too!!

To continue; when she mentioned his first name, I said, "I know him, his dad gave me my very first professional haircut, when I was three years old, in Bonnyville, Alberta!" I was correct!

On another coincidental note, we had our wedding at the same Church, exactly six years later (yep same date), with the same Minister. You won't believe this; however, I was the one that chose the wedding invitations, to which Beth approve, and unbeknownst to either of us, until commented on by her friend, the invitations were the exact same invitations that her dear friend had chosen for their wedding. What can I say, we were meant to be!!!

27 APRIL, 2018

It was Beth's Birthday on the 24th of April, and I now reflect on our situation.

I don't want to trivialize any other known Disease. I cannot imagine the horror of being locked in a condition where you have absolutely no control over your body, and yet have full mental awareness, you might say the opposite of Alzheimer's. I cannot fathom going through the deterioration of MS, or Parkinson's, or Palsy. To develop a heart disease can either end suddenly, or a lifetime of medication and monitoring, either way, extremely hard on the patient, and/or the family.

And Cancer! Undoubtably one of the most feared, and painful of all diseases! You first go into shock and disbelief that you have been diagnosed with Cancer; then the potential treatment, which is the harshest in all of humanity; then the prognosis, even with that being as 'Terminal', there is a sliver of hope, still, most assuredly, the certainty of pain!

With these, and many other diseases, there are occurrences of hope, denial, and eventually acceptance! With Alzheimer's, there is no cure, there is no reprieve, there is no hope! All there is, is instant acceptance that it will end in death; be it five years or twenty! There are minor ups and downs; however, the deterioration is constant, and linear! There are dips where you panic, and feel a sense of fear that the end is quickly closing in, and then, reprieve back to the norm of regression and depression! Regression that keeps going backwards down the growth cycle of life! A once vibrant, brilliant, loving adult regress into childhood, to the point of birth; with the opposite result, death!

Trust me, I would not wish for, or trade, Alzheimer's for any other disease. Suffering for Beth is minimal...only confusion and anxiety. I am fortunate to be in a position where I can devote my entire time to being with Beth, not everyone has the luxury of being able to do that. Many people have jobs that must be performed, children to attend to, duties that must be fulfilled.

At this juncture, all I can say is that there is no guilt that should be assimilated by anyone! All you can do, is the best you can. My current duties, and abilities, are to make sure I spend every possible moment with Beth. I feel like I am growing old with her, which is the dream of every newlywed... for now, I am fortunate!!

MOTHERHOOD

6 JUNE 2018

You have never seen a more beautiful sight! The precious person lays before you, and you beam with love. As she sleeps, her small fingers hold on to your thumb as if life depended on it, and you don't want to leave. In fact, you want to embrace this precious moment forever! You gaze upon her curly hair, and her beautiful features; you pray for nothing except for the best for this precious parcel.

The care and attention this person needs is overwhelming, and you treasure every moment of it. The feeding, the cleaning, the anxiety of not knowing what she needs or when she needs it, the dedication is all worth it! You treasure every moment as you try to communicate, and though the sounds are incomprehensible, the smiles melt your heart to the core.

It is at this moment in time that, as much as a man can, I truly understand motherhood!! I stand in awe as I look down upon this child that was once my spouse.

Anticipation of the vision of what is to come is replaced with the tears of depression; of the vision of what has transpired! All your fears are now realized!!

PERSONALITY THEFT

4 AUGUST, 2018

I'm talking about Alzheimer's, and the patient! Alzheimer's takes away your 'Free Will', robing you of choice. Choice of food, drink, where to go, what to wear, what to do, where to live and even what to say. Worst thing to happen, is to also lose your personality, the essence of who you are.

Time/Life relationship. 'Time' becomes a function of thought; 'Life' becomes a function of time. There is no past or future. Your memories become the 'Present', the 'Past' is where you live, and there is no tomorrow. She knows she has a son, and yet can't understand where he is. She was bathing him a few moments ago as a child… where did he go? "Today, my son is eighteen months old!" (not forty-five and standing beside her); "I don't have a daughter Jenny!" (She hasn't been born yet); "Shall we go for a walk tomorrow?" (a question you will never more be asked, nor be able to satisfy).

With Alzheimer's you also start to lose your communication skills. Forgetting how to express what you want to say, formulating coherency in what you are trying to say. Self-expression gives away to simply trying to say anything. Comprehending others is strained until eventually, all they do is ask you the same questions; "Don't you know who I am?"; "Why don't you remember me?".

THREE WAY PERSPECTIVE

There are three ways to look at how Alzheimer's will change your life. Yes, now this is about you!!

The first way you can look at it, is how it will change her life. With this perspective, you will feel sorry for her, curse the world, and all that is in it… perhaps even the heavens. Do a lot of crying, and feel remorse over what she could do, and cannot do anymore; what she loved, and what she is now oblivious to; the memories that were, and the memories now lost; essentially, what she was, and what she is turning into. You will live in a long-lasting world of grief!

The second way to perceive the effects this illness will have; is how it will affect you. Eventually, no more camping, fishing, travelling; essentially, no more recreation. There is also all the work you will have to do like, washing dishes, washing clothes, cleaning the house, making the beds, even cook all the meals. Then there is taking care of her! This my friend includes dressing her, feeding her your cooking (hope it's not a new experience for her), bathing her, and eventually, toileting her. And at the deepest level, 'Sex'! How will you survive without 'Sex'?? The horror of it all!

Of course, when she forgets who you are, you will feel like all is lost. All this will be a new experience for her as well, and you may just find some resistance that will drive you to the edge!!! "Man, this is such an inconvenience!" "This is hell!!"

But the third way of handling this tragedy, is to look at how she perceives this disease is affecting her. She starts to forget the simple things, like how to dress, how to eat, how to clean the mess you are making (trust me this one is a big issue for her), even to the point of how to go to the toilet. Now imagine yourself in this position, as being diagnosed with Alzheimer's; you can't fix things around the house, can't fix the car, heck, they won't even let you drive anymore!! "What the hell is going on??" "I'm so confused!!"

Like I said, those are the simple things. Now let's think of how she feels not remembering people, even her own husband and children. How embarrassing it must be when you're expected to know all these strange people. Some old guy says he's your husband, and your husband is only twenty-six years old! "Is this all a cruel joke?" Next thing you know, strange people are dressing and undressing you, taking your clothes off, and sitting you on the throne. What they do to you when you're done is unmentionable!! In fact, it's horrific!!

You will experience all three perspectives, and the path you choose to handle such situations will be based on one of these perspectives…choose carefully!! The one you choose will affect both the rest of your relationship, and the rest of your life. How much do you love her? What is her worth to you? Unfortunately, many people opt out of caring because of the inconvenience! If so, God help you if you should end up in the same boat.

THE FINAL DAYS

They allowed me to feed Beth all the time. I knew the end was near when I would feed Beth the puree, and it would simply drool out of her mouth. Soon she started to choke; her mind could no longer process the function of swallowing food and water, the essentials of life.

What can I do? I asked the Health Care Nurse that very question; the answer pounded on my heart like an eighteen pound sledge hammer… "Nothing!" It seemed unrealistic, there must be something that could be done. I realize it was as hard on the Health Care Nurse as it was for me, regrettably, the answer was definitive. The only unthinkable alternative was force feeding and hydration… not acceptable!!

"Nothing!" was not the exact word or words, and sounds like a callus response of a heartless dictator; the opposite was true. Truthfully, that was all my feeble, remorseful mind could comprehend. I couldn't bear the thought of Beth suffering from hunger and thirst.

This wonderful, caring person consoled me in that, although Beth could no longer function in her own survival, she would not suffer. She would be given Morphine to ease her suffering while transitioning from the bonds of life, and crossing over Jordan. "How long?" "Hard to say, could be three days, could be two weeks." And now for the great unknown, what do I do in the interim? There was no validity in justifying my meager existence by just sitting back, and watching. Many people have gone through this before, and I can now empathize with them; my world was about to end!!! You simply cannot understand the futility of the situation; the thought was brutal!!!

It's a proven fact that sound is one of the last of the senses to be extinguished. I firmly believe that God has allowed hearing to be the last sense to go for a reason. All I could think of, was to keep talking to her, and play music for her constantly. Through my grief, my calm and reassuring voice was necessary, reassuring that "all would be ok", akin to the last lie I would constantly have to tell Beth. The one time in my life when lies didn't matter, white or black.

I was determined to be there for Beth's last breath; however, with the uncertainty of time, I needed to eat, sleep, and be able to remain positive for my sweetheart. Every night, before I left, her vitals were taken to see what progression, or more accurately regression, was taking place. At the end of the tenth day, her vitals were confirmed as still being strong… at five o'clock in the morning I received the fateful call… Beth was no longer with us!!!

Though we lived four blocks away from the continuing care centre, in what seemed like seconds, I was with her. It was hard to realize she was not breathing, and yet somehow, I was relieved. Her suffering was over! There was nothing more I could do!! I took her into my arms for one last time to relive the memory of our bond with a final hug. It felt so reassuring and familiar in that her body was still warm, the memory, and the feeling of which, will carry me until I reunite with her. "Goodbye my Love, till we meet again!!"

This is where it all falls in!!! The culmination of a love lost; the vortex of life!! Nothing, and I mean nothing, matters to you anymore. If you don't believe in the afterlife, you pray you are wrong.

And now the guilt!! Maybe some of the guilt stems from me wanting to be there with her as she took her last breath; and yet not being there. Guilt is an emotion that I fail to rationalize, and I feel compelled to reveal more on my insecurity, relating to my feeling of 'guilt', in a section further in this book.

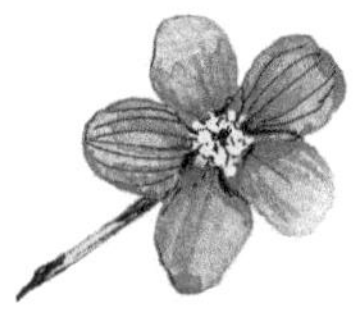

Chapter: The Eulogy/Obituary!

21 SEPT, 2018

Beth fell asleep last night. God came by, and took her hand; she is now at rest. Don't feel sad for Beth or me, because we are both at Peace. Following is the Obituary that was created by our son and daughter-in-law, and printed in the local paper.

DOROTHY ELIZABETH BLAIS

Following a seven-year battle with Alzheimer's, Dorothy Elizabeth Blais, known to friends and family as Beth, passed away peacefully September 21, 2018 at the age of seventy-one.

A wife, mother, sister, and friend, Beth will be remembered as a loving, kind woman who always had a smile on her face, a mischievous twinkle in her eye, and never refused a hug. Whether sharing laughs with friends or family around a campfire, or dancing the night away with her husband, Beth loved life, and truly cherished the special people who were part of it.

She is survived and mourned by her one true love, husband Arthur, who was by her side throughout. Grieving her passing are her mother, father-in-law, son, daughter-in-Law, and grandsons. Also mourning her loss are brothers, sisters-in-law, as well as numerous nieces and nephews, and close friends.

The family also wishes to thank the wonderful staff of the Westlock Continuing Care Centre for making Beth's final days comfortable.

If I could ever have just one more day and wishes did come true,
I'd spend every glorious moment side by side with you.
Recalling all the years we shared and the memories we made,
How grateful I would be to have just one more day.
Where the tears I shed are not in vain and only fall in bliss,
So many things I'd let you know about the days you've missed.
I wouldn't have to make pretend you never went away,
How grateful I would be to have just one more day.
When that day came to a close and the sun began to set,
A million times I'd let you know I never will forget.
The heart of gold you left behind when you entered Heaven's gate,
How grateful I would be to have just one more day.

FUNERAL/CELEBRATION OF LIFE

Many people gather at elaborate funerals with their friends and family to honour the dearly departed soul, that is the accepted custom. When Beth's stepfather passed away, he instructed that there would be no funeral service on his passing, unconscionable, and yet…!!

Beth and I discussed our passing, and realized this was more in line with what we wanted for our demise. The thought of our friends and family sitting in different corners of the room, sobbing and grieving was unbearable. Meeting and greeting the survivor with pity in their eyes would only make things worse. Neither of us wanted to put the ones we cherished in that position.

DON'T GET ME WRONG! Closure is very important to some, and funerals are a means to provide that. I'm not against funerals at all, it's just that it wasn't for Beth and I. As such, the thought of a funeral was not in our cards, better to just leave quietly; Wake be damned, we shared a lot of revelry with our friends when we were alive and together, those are the memories we wanted to live on.

On behalf of Beth's passing, our dear and beloved daughter-in-law found a beautiful farewell message, and created a memorial package, which consisted of an envelope, tied to a handmade card, with a pretty, little, purple flower glued on the upper right corner, and an inscription saying;

You are so very special
I wanted you to know
And as a way to remember
I've sent these seeds to sow
Plant them in your garden
Or in a pretty pot
And as the flowers start to bloom
Please forget me not

In Loving Memory of Beth Blais

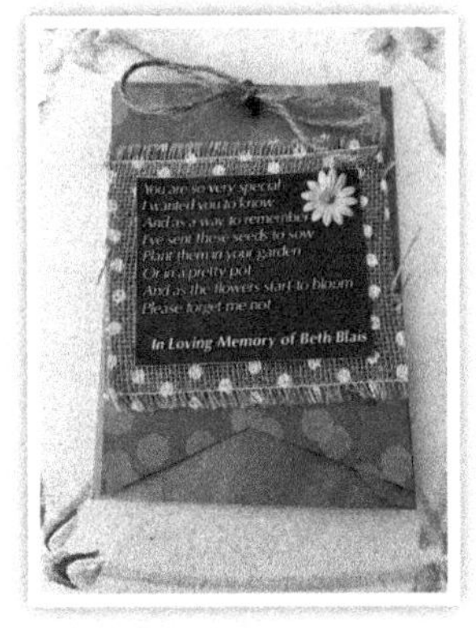

Inside the envelope, a package of 'Forget-Me-Not' seeds!

In leu of a funeral, and as a 'Celebration of Life', I made it a point to personally visit all our friends and family, and deliver these cards by hand; to those I missed, I apologize!

The gathering of our friends' and relatives' together, in the comfort of their homes, was personal and wonderful! We were able to relive cherished memories of Beth together, on a one-on-one basis, in a relaxed environment. The experience was amazing, and a memory I will cherish forever. I cannot think of a more befitting and personal manner to say "Goodbye"!!

When Beth was cremated, I requested a miniature urn and a cross pendent containing some of her ashes. I also designed, and went under the needles of a tattoo artist (something I said I would never do) as a lasting memorial to the release of the grip of Alzheimer's, and to the love I feel for this blessed soul! It depicts a purple ribbon as a symbol of Alzheimer's, the inside of the ribbon in the shape of a red heart, all cradled by a set of Angel's wings, depicting her accent into heaven. When I travel, Beth comes with me!

This is time for another financial consideration you must be aware of, and this one hit me hard. Not only did I not consider funeral expenses, which were an added burden, what hit me the hardest was that after Beth passed away, her pension was transferred over to me as the surviving spouse. What didn't occur to me at the time, was that Beth was a dependent of sorts, and that her taxes were separate from mine. Result was that as I went from a married status to a single marital status; I was catapulted into the next tax bracket, and last year I owed $6,995 in back taxes. OUCH!!! I wasn't ready for that, and subjected to pay within three months.

By the time Beth passed away, I was broke! I didn't have any savings; I didn't have any investment, and I had debts to pay. Because of the cost of care, amongst all the other expenses, I didn't have any money available to pay $6,995 back! The Taxation Department must think I suddenly became a millionaire when in reality I make below the national average family income!! $6,995 divided by 12 means my pension just went down by $582.91 per month, and as I didn't revise the tax being withheld automatically till late last year, I will owe an additional $3,497.50 this year. This sucks!! Be advised, and consider this carefully!!

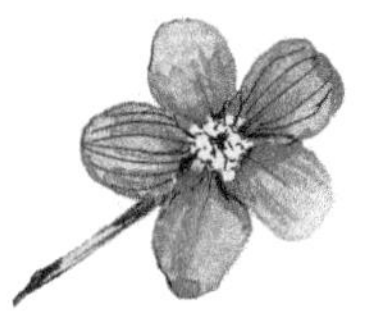

Chapter: Sexuality

There is one thing that you will find sorely lacking in this book, sexuality. I realize that is probably the most pertinent and important questions some of you would like to have answered, unfortunately that is something I can't help you with very much.

It is documented that every patient will react differently with their sexuality, ranging from complete disassociation, to displaying disinhibited behaviors. You will have to assess your own situation in particular. As for myself, I felt that engaging in intimacy would be considered as taking advantage of someone that was incapable of deciding for themselves. Forcing myself on Beth would have been unconscionable.

One thing I need to clarify is that it wasn't Beth that failed to engage in sexuality, it was me. Beth was always a very sensual lover, and our interactions were fantastic. About two years before Beth developed Alzheimer's my libido turned left, and went South.

I saw the Doc about it, and tests revealed that my testosterone levels were in fact down, not significantly although at a noticeable level. I was subsequently prescribed testosterone to help boost my libido. After about six months on a regiment, further tests revealed there was no difference. I even looked for, and tried the holistic and organic approach; unfortunately, to no avail. It could have simply been a mineral deficiency; however, the doctor should have picked that one up.

Within the pages of this book, I often reflect on 'Divine Intervention', and maybe this was God's way of preparing me for the inevitable; sexuality with Beth was not to be in the cards, perhaps for a good reason.

I know it may sound hokey to some of you; however, if you have patience with me, I will try to provide you with something to consider that is very important. OK, I just mentioned 'Divine Intervention', and this is my reasoning. Perhaps the good Lord was providing his influence on *both* of us for Beth's benefit.

Consider this, I was influenced by having my libido striped away years before Beth developed Alzheimer's. The potential reason being, that my moral fibre would not allow me to take advantage of Beth in her condition, as I previously mentioned. My lack of sex drive allowed me to focus on her health, wellbeing, and acclimation into a world confused by the cultural attributes of modern society. My need for sexual fulfilment was diminished throughout this arduous transition in Beth's life. The normal sex drive is strong, yet my requirements were minimal.

And now for the flip side, and what matters most. I feel the good Lord understands what goes on in a confused mind of an Alzheimer's patient. There are two things to consider; firstly, I mentioned disinhibited behaviour in the beginning paragraphs of this chapter. If we would have had normal drives and encounters, up to and during this infliction, once the moral fibre I referred to earlier would have taken over, Beth would have seemingly been 'cut off'. Now I don't have to tell you what that feels like, I'm sure we've all been subject to this at some point or another. For Beth, in her confused state of mind, and being the sensual and sexual person she was, being 'cut off' would have been a traumatic event predicating anxiety, with no way of expressing the anguish. In her diminished communication capability, how could she have questioned, "What did I do wrong?" "Don't you love me anymore?" "Are you cheating on me?" All things that would go through a normal mindset.

Secondly, and this is something to consider seriously! The mind of an Alzheimer's patient transitions constantly to a different time and place in an instant. Today, all is normal, or so it seems, you are sitting beside her when she asks where her husband is, "We're on our honeymoon, and I can't find him." "Who the heck are you?" Don't laugh, it happens!! Now consider if this happens while you are making love to her… "My God! Help! I'm being Raped!!" Not laughing anymore, are you??

This is my reasoning for believing in 'Divine Intervention'! I firmly believe that the good Lord, in all his wisdom, helped us transition; me into celibacy, and Beth into lowered expectations. It worked like a charm!! Beth and I had no negative encounters, and her Alzheimer's progressed with little, if any, anxiety. God must have loved his special angle very much, and I am so thankful!!

And now I revert the focus onto yourself. What should you do? I can't tell you that because my experience and perception, will be vastly different than any of you. Is it OK to have continued intimacy? Morally and physiologically… probably; however, I can assure you I am no expert in these matters!

I don't suggest that she be 'cut off', as it were; however, your expectations of sex must change. I can only suggest that you focus more on her reaction to every encounter, and less of your satisfaction as a need. This may be new to you; nonetheless, if you've been experiencing a fantastic mutual relationship throughout your union, you understand of which I speak; her needs before yours!! I assume there will come a time when she questions what is going on, and that must be considered as a sign of the time for things to change. God help both of you!!

And now I must return to my experience for clarity.

Regarding being intimate after the diagnosis, we did have an encounter shortly after Beth had been diagnosed, and all I can say is that the experience had changed. The encounter was missing an important element, the lack of sensuality. Beth was a willing participant, yet she responded in a reactive manner, with seemingly no intimacy whatsoever; it was purely a responsive gesture. I don't blame Beth whatsoever, how could I? It's possible Alzheimer's could have already permeated the portion of the brain that controls intimacy.

Most likely, her brain is occupied with the constructs of confusion and anxiety, probably not on thoughts of sensuality.

I want to make it perfectly clear that this in no way affected my love for Beth. I held her in the highest admiration, and was always so happy to be with her. I beamed with pride when we were with friends, or in a public setting. There were always a lot of meaningful hugs and kisses together towards the end; remorsefully, just not a lot of sensuality. I feel that my neglect of onus in the sexuality department, is one of the major aspects that perpetuates and enhances my feeling of remorse. Did I not fulfill her desires? I wish I could have known!!!

Again, what advice can I provide? It's totally up to you; nonetheless, I feel that sensuality must be mutual. Your need for sex may be a strong driver, and only you can determine what's more important, your fulfilment, or her need for compassion, empathy, love, and perhaps, sexuality.

Extra Marital affairs? I would never consider it, and I suggest it is not a good idea. After seeing Beth in her final stages, and feeling the ultimate love I have for this lady, the shame and disappointment I would feel with myself, would be unbearable. The feeling of love that flourishes in the final stages, was a level of love I can only hope you achieve as well. A sense of love I can only compare to that of a when you have a newly born child, which in essence, your spouse gradually becomes. The level of anguish I now feel, after going through this juncture in life, is unrelenting, and would have been far too much to cope with if I had strayed.

My level of sexuality now??? I have no idea!

CARETAKER HANGOVER

You know, I thought once Beth had passed away it would be over. Yes, I expected there would be a couple years of mourning, grief, and self-pity, after which I could just move on with my life…not so fast Bunckie!!! Take heed my friend, grief, and in my case guilt, are neither easy, quick, nor avoidable to deal with.

The rest of this book has no relevance regarding Alzheimer's, and how it affected Beth; nonetheless, I felt it relevant to keep documenting what was impacting me, as my journey was far from over. Perhaps you can benefit from my experiences.

What happens next is rather lengthy, emotional, and fret with pitfalls pertaining to the experience you might subject yourself to after you lose the love of your life. It is tragic, overwhelming, and requires support. It is my account of what I went through, and I welcome you to keep reading while your loved one is still alive. Perhaps you'll be prepared for a world of grief, or to cope with the understanding that what you are, or might be, experiencing as being normal.

Actually, it's not all bad, or doesn't have to be bad at all. I overheard Garth Brooks, a famous 'Country and Western' singer (I'm old, and don't know what they call the modern-day genre for his type of music) while listening to his Sirius XM Station, talking about his father regarding his mom's passing. Though not exact, his words of relevance were, "There are two ways people handle the death of their spouse. Either you pick up the pieces, and move on, or you build a Shrine in their honour… my dad built a Shrine!" As you will no doubt see in the following pages of this book, I'm not sure where I stand.

Through observation, I have always thought that the worst thing you can do is fall into a 'Rebound Relationship'. I swore that that would never happen to me; little did I realize the grieving process that goes on after the loss of someone you love. It matters little if the loss is through the death of your partner, or even just the demise of a relationship through divorce. There are many occurrences of a quick re-marriage, followed by a quick divorce, or worse, a continued life of regret.

Of course, this is personal, and different for everyone, yet still relevant. I never thought I would fall for it, and guess what?? No, I didn't get married! I fell into what can best be described as 'Caregiver Hangover'… sort of like, 'a bit of the hair of the dog that bit you'… it eases your pain for now, still, you know you will suffer for it later.

After seven years of imposed isolation from society, while taking care of Beth, and devoting all my time to her care, I found it familiar, and easy to carry on with the lifestyle I had now grown accustomed to. The solution at hand, was to continue to care for someone else, and thereby relieving me of the guilt of getting into a rebound relationship, and forsaking my love for Beth. I felt she would approve of this transition in my life, not realizing that caregiving, at times, can evolve into the familiarity of a lasting, loving relationship. I could easily summarize this effect, and end the book right now; believe me, it's far too complex to just skim over. Stay tuned in folks, more on that to come.

I again must fall back on continuing the timeline approach. I follow with a rather lengthy account of my thoughts and feelings which has presided over the course of this entire book; an account that many of you will consider 'Hogwash'; nevertheless, the journey continues.

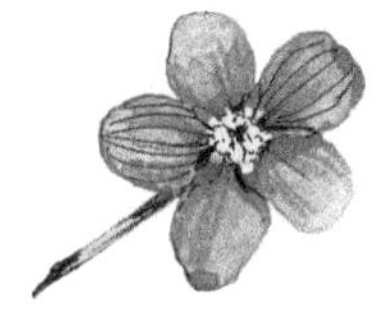

Chapter: Post-mortem

28TH OCTOBER, 2018

As mentioned above, after the onset of arrangements to be taken care of, I traveled to many of our relatives and friends, to distribute the Celebration of Life packages in Beth's memory. There were many wishes of condolences relayed in both directions, and the packages were well appreciated. A special thanks to my daughter-in-law!! I found the travelling to be a great form of distraction, interspersed with time of solitude on the road, filled with sad music, and tears.

I felt it was a befitting time to grieve, so I thought a longer trip would be in order as a time of reflection. Beth and I had talked about wanting to take a trip through Route 66, so I planned such a trip to fulfill a desire we both had, taking her with me in absentia. I have a niece in Toronto, to which I could deliver a Celebration of Life package, and conveniently, I could also deliver all the effects she left behind in Edmonton, when she left five years previously, as further justification. It was the perfect excuse to go East, and then head to Chicago, and hop on the beginning of 'the Mother Road'. The time was right weatherwise, as we were not yet in the throes of Winter, so my destiny was at hand.

2 NOV, 2018

Leaving Chicago, and towards the beginning of my escapade through Route 66 after Beth's passing, I stopped at one of the many tourist attractions lining this famous Route called the 'Gemini Giant' in Wilmington, Illinois. It stands outside the 'Launching Pad Drive-in Restaurant'. There I discovered the owners, Tully Garrett and Holly Barker, had purchased the attraction just over a year before, and have begun refurbishing the property, and restaurant.

I found the owners of the establishment to be warm and friendly, and after I told them about the purpose for my trip, they told me they got together after the loss of their respective spouses. In dealing with their grief, they formed an association called 'Grief Anonymous' Facebook Group. I joined the forum, and have found a lot of support from the people going through this juncture in life called 'Grief'. They are still active, and I encourage you to seek out this forum on Facebook, as a source of support.

11 NOV, 2018

Sad day! Beth's brother, Brian, passed away from complications with Alzheimer's. He developed Phenomena while in the Calgary Hospital Care Centre. He had been diagnosed with Alzheimer's only about 6 months prior, and went quickly. This was quite unexpected, and my trip will be terminated shortly.

My intension was to complete Route 66, and follow the coastline highway up California, Oregon, and Washington; however, with the California wildfires in progress, and the urgency to return, I will start my return home in a few days when I reach the end of the Route, as completion of this trip.

16 NOV, 2018

End of the road… no, not for me, the end of Route 66 on the Santa Monica Pier. Felt I needed to finish the trip with Beth. Found it quite touching, and had a picture taken with me holding Beth's miniature Urn under the 'End of Route 66' Sign. Tears did flow.

The intent of this trip for me, was to provide a distraction, and some isolation to help me come to terms with Beth's passing; something I thought should be done in privacy, and not shared. We had discussed on many occasions how our passing should be, and just slipping away was the intent, that's how Beth would have wanted it for herself.

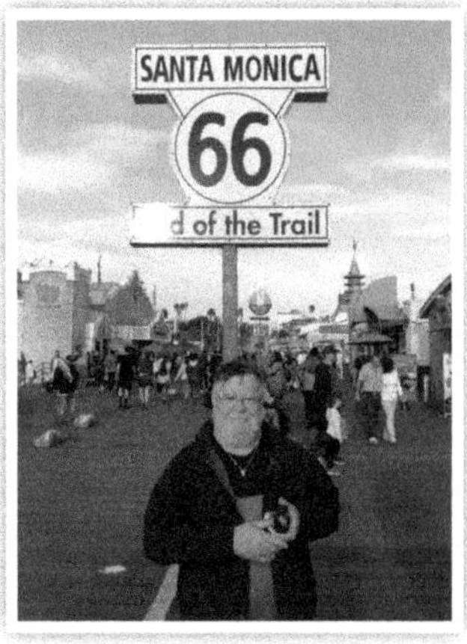

In saying that, I realize that this trip ended up being the exact opposite of what was intended of our wishes, sorry Beth! The distraction helped me to accept my loss; however, the reality was that my grief, rekindled cherished memories of my loved one. I can't think of a better way of providing some closure I needed over Beth's passing. I'd like to think that whenever I encounter anything in relation to Route 66, I'll remember this journey, and Beth, with happy and fond memories.

23 NOV, 2018

The objective was met yesterday in the completion of Route 66, and I am returning home. It's a journey that Beth and I had talked about doing before things got crazy. The tears I referred to on the Santa Monica Pier, was an outcome that I did not expect. I guess it unwittingly represented the end of two journeys, and it saddened me so. It does not mean, by any means, that the grieving process is complete, much the opposite I suspect.

I thought it would be easier for me. I thought that seeing Beth go from the vibrant, intelligent, fun, and loving person she was, and regressing to the state of a newborn child over the course of seven years, had allowed me to grieve over time. It's been like looking at each other through a one-way mirror where her opacity increased to a point where I no longer existed in her eyes. It digs a hole in your heart that just increases with time. I consoled myself in that she was my whole purpose in life, it wasn't about me, it was all about her…suddenly, it's all about me!

I miss being with Beth so much. My son was so right in his obituary saying "If I could have just one more day" where she could smile at me and say, "it's all right!". That's all I need!! I was with her to the end; however, I feel I never got to say goodbye to her. More so, I never got to hear her say goodbye to me… and now she's gone, and the pain is real!

FEB 28, 2019 TO COSTA RICA

So, there I was, at my kid's place, babysitting their Dog, and two cats while they are in Palm Springs California. This is one week after I spent a week dog sitting my sister's dog while they were in Mexico! It's -32 C, and I'm out there walking the dog when it hits me… What the Hell?? I'm retired, have no commitments, able to travel at the drop of a hat, and here I am, dog sitting in the cold while they're enjoying the warmth of anyplace other than here!! What's wrong with this picture??? That's when I decided "That's it, I'm outa here!!"

Oh yeah!!! I remember why I don't like to fly, and I forgot the basic rule!! Note to self, 'Pack Light!!'… and the fun begins. So, I had Homeland Security scratching their heads, I brought some of Beth's ashes in the miniature Urn I mentioned before; she is free of any drug suspicions… me on the other hand… I got the evil eye!

GOD'S WAKE-UP CALL

I'm in Huston on a 6-hour layover, and I've had a few rums so here's a revelation for you; God talked to me last night, I just wish I knew what he was saying. Mind you, that's how God always works.

I was having a restless dream of an ever-recurrent vision that, of course, didn't make sense. Basically, there was a pool of water (or a lake), and at times, people surrounded by what can best be explained as a bag full of air; something like a bunch of people in an inflatable lifeboat. The dilemma I faced was to either pull, and move the raft with people, to the edge to safety, or get inside, and enjoy the party (they were all having fun). There was no threat or requirement to move them, nevertheless, it was a potential task to complete. Then, just before I woke up at 3:00 a.m. plain as day, everything stopped. Once awake, I sensed I HAD a choice to make!

Interpretation of dreams are always ambiguous at best; mine translated into "do I want to jump in, and join the party, or move it out of the way, and move on!" I related that as, "do I want to die, join Beth, and be happy, or be satisfied that all is well, and get on with the rest of my life?" I chose life!! I've only got one life to live, just as well find out what's in store! What strikes me as relevant, is that I was distinctively given a choice, one that wasn't decided during my dream; awake, I made a firm decision!!

Now obviously everyone's perceptions will be different, and we each will read something into this dream, regardless, it was my dream.

God I miss my Beth!! The loneliness, the emptiness, the void I feel is mine to bear, and all about me. It seems self-serving, and yet, I don't care about myself, I care about myself without Beth; the one thing…the only thing…in my life I wouldn't change, even to her death…even to my death.

15 MAR, 2019 RETURN FROM COSTA RICA

21 MAR, 2019

So, you think you have it rough! You ain't seen nothing yet!!

It's been almost 6 months since Beth's 'Passing Over', and the last two days have been the hardest! Just came back from a two-week vacation to Costa Rica, which was OK. It was a nice get-away. Now that I'm back, old haunts are getting to me. In the last two days, Beth is first and foremost in my mind. Every song I hear, every silence I face, every diversion I take, brings me back to her. I tried the old tried and true, and…Nada! My rum quota has been exceeded for the day.

I guess my thoughts keep coming back to communication. Where I currently live, I don't have many friends close by, and the potential for meaningful relationship, companionship, is nil. I really don't feel like hanging around with the Coffee group, I don't really know anyone, and have absolutely nothing in common with them. I did drive a Cockshut Tractor once; needless to say, I'm sure that wouldn't impress them too much. I have all sorts of friends I can associate with; however, with them all I can relive in my mind is the past with Beth. Did we have a good time together? You bet-ya!! Was Beth a big part of our friendship?? You know it. Can I plan a future with my friends?? Not at all! They have their lives, and I'm just a visitor! Can I discover a new meaning of life? It seems pointless without Beth!

All I want to do is be able to talk to someone, maybe about their kids, grandkids, their marriage, their husband, whatever!! I need someone to allow me to experience life as they feel it…mine right now is the shits!! I don't want them to bear my children, nor have them make lifelong commitments; all I want is to relive a normal life. My life was great; nevertheless, that door was closed six months ago! Right now, life consists of sad memories, and occasional rum (and it's not working).

I sat outside in the wonderful sun this afternoon, while a potato and a carrot caramelized on the BBQ. Then, I slapped a steak on the BBQ, and cooked it to perfection! Now, what kind of man can't appreciate that? While stuffing my face, and thinking of Beth, I got an attack of some sort; suspect it was anxiety. What happened is that I was thinking about Beth, and how much she would have enjoyed this supper, then suddenly, I couldn't take in a breath! I couldn't breathe! Not through my mouth, nor through my nose. I went into meditation mode, and eventually I was able to breathe through my mouth. Took what seemed like an eternity before I could take a good breath through my nose! Right now, life sucks, and I assume it will suck for you too.

There's no easy way to grieve and move on. Everybody's life is different, and you might fare well. All I know is I thought I was tough, and thought that I would be able to move on with the knowledge that I did everything I could to ease her transition. When it was over, I wouldn't have to worry about her anymore, and I would be relieved. I didn't count on missing her so much, and for so long. I have no ambition to replace her, I just want to remember her, and enjoy the memories of the good times we had. Well, I hope you're stronger than I am, because the loneliness, and the vacuum she left behind hurts more than you can imagine! Screw it, I'm having another rum!!!

29 MARCH, 2019

I do have a friend that I talk to frequently; unfortunately, her problems far outweigh anything I can come up with. We have become good friends, and I feel privileged to be able to console her when she needs my shoulder, and vice versa.

Anne was Beth's next-door resident at the continuing care centre. Anne had a very close relationship with a man named Gilles, the love of her life!! They both were wheelchair bound; Anne with MS, and Gilles with more debilitating and painful diseases than I can name. As they were both of French lineage, he would often speak to her with a French, 'Pepe-Le-Pew' accent, "Come with me! I will take you to de Kasbah, and we will dance the night away, hon-hon!!".

He loved Anne with his whole heart and soul for eight years! June 2018, he died of what was eventually ruled an accidental overdose, even now, something Anne blames herself for. She believes he committed suicide, and it was her fault because the day before he died, she told him that they were through! Her reasoning was that she didn't want him to see her deteriorate as the MS progressed.

When she mentioned Gilles' passing to me in June, she was in a severely traumatized mental state! Firstly, she thought he committed suicide because of her, and secondly, as a former Catholic, she figured he would be sent into the damnation of Hell, and they could never be reunited. She told me she was considering suicide as well. She needed someone to talk to, so I befriended her. We had both been in the military, so we had a natural bond, and were able to confide in each other.

At some point in time, she said that I reminded her so much of Gilles, which she continually repeated, and I appreciate to this day. I felt honoured to be thought of in this manner, and being of French descent myself, would do the Pepe-Le-Pew thing for her.

Alas, I now must transition our friendship into reality before this gets out of hand. I remind her of Gilles, and she refers to me as such; however, I am not Gilles! Gilles will always be her soulmate, and she must differentiate between the two of us. I want her to be happy in the memories of Gilles, and that we are, and will remain good friends.

For my part, I have been on antidepressants for the last six years, and they have worked well…too well! My whole trip on Route 66 was meant as a distraction to grieve, instead, each day was filled with humorous misadventures. I am weening myself off them slowly, and now realize they have prevented me from grieving. I knew there was something wrong because since Beth's death, I have been emotionally all over the place! I'm walking around, smiling from ear to ear, as if I'm happy she passed away, and when asked if I'm doing ok? "Just fine!!" Then I turn the corner or hear a song, and while I'm alone, the water works start! I do not have a water retention problem! That's where Anne has been so close to my heart, because I can cry with her.

But I digress! I'm not alright, I'm badly bent! At times I think of being with other women, and in the same moment in time, I grieve over losing Beth; the guilt hits me like a brick! I'm a social being, and I want so much to hold Beth again, that sometimes I just want someone, anyone, in my arms, again with impending guilt.

That is my reasoning for getting off antidepressants! Gradually, I'm realizing that I don't want to be with anyone else, as of yet. I just want to think of the times Beth and I were together, and be able to smile. I still have a lot of grieving to do!

10 JULY, 2019

I haven't mentioned this before; however, out of a need for a distraction I bought a Motorcycle a while ago… not a Harley, though that would have been nice, a cheap plastic Japanese make. My intention was to determine if I wanted to get into the biking lifestyle, as a means to an end… that being, continued distractions.

I made the decision to leave for Vancouver Island for a bike trip; so, I loaded the bike in the trailer, and waved goodbye. Purpose for my trip was to visit friends, scope out a potential place to live, and just feel the freedom of hopping on a bike, and just ride; I was not disappointed.

It was a great visit with great friends; nevertheless, there was something missing… or someone! Don't get me wrong, enjoyed the visit but there wasn't much going on. As always, all good things must come to an end! I was planning to stay another week, the biking was good; unfortunately, the weather was socking in with a lot of wet stuff, not particularly good for biking. I have mentioned that I'm not a Bad Ass, Hard Core Biker Dude yet, haven't I? Or at least, 'I'm too old for this Shit'! Seems that the latter was the theme of this trip.

Anyways, that was till yesterday! I've got three Navigation Units that comes with my Mazda: Apple Maps, Google Maps, and Mazda Nav GPS. The only reason I'm mentioning this, is that my Google Maps GPS did something totally out of character! I was dumbstruck (I mean more than usual)! On my way back, I decided to go through our old haunts at Gull Lake (where Beth and I used to live, for those that don't know). Beth and I used to just hop in a vehicle, and explore back country roads just for the whim of it. As I got closer to Rimbey, the memory of our exploits came pouring back with every road I recognized in passing. The memories just got more vivid, and the thought of never being able to relive those memories with Beth became unbearable!! There wasn't a dry eye in the car (sorry to my Rimbey friends, I just couldn't drop in)!

Again, I digress! My memories seem to permeate with fits of the loss; back to the GPS quirk! North of Bentley, I turned right, off HWY 20 onto HWY 771. The Google GPS said, "go North 600 Meters, and turn left to get back onto HWY 20". I knew where I was going. Being upset, I hollered, "F*^k Off!!!" Believe it or not, I'll swear on Beth's ashes, it listened!! Beth and I found about 5 different ways to get to Edmonton, and for the rest of my return trip, the GPS would intuitively choose the direction I was deciding to take 'ahead of time'; regardless of how indirect or longer it was. It would also hi-light an alternate way I could redirect without saying a word… most notably, the voice guidance was not muted! Nothing was said, you know, the usual "Recalculating, turn left, bla, bla, bla!!" Nothing like this has ever happened to me before, and probably will never happen again!! Needless to say, I feel God, and Beth, were taking pity on me that day!

So now I'm home! Walk in the door, and there it was… my rum collection with more rum than I will ever drink!! My couch, my beautiful, cozy couch! And my toilet, the perfect height, with my comfortable, soft closing seat! And my TP! OMG, my TP, with man sized, soft, absorbent sheets (note to self: never leave home without it again!). My bed! My how I've missed you as I lay on your soft comfort top like floating on a cloud… flying above the trees… in a rocking chair… with Max at my… ZzzZzzZzz

20 JULY, 2019 (TOO SOON OLD!)

I aged very quickly in the last couple weeks. The despondency of an old fart is taking over. At one time we had it all! Now there's nothing that matters. They say, "It's not the destination, it's the journey!" For me, I am 'destination challenged', and the journey is only time wasted from point 'A' to point 'B'. Back to grieving Beth.

25 JULY, 2019

Involved in 'Sadness Therapy' today. Went to a weekly event at the 'Blues on Whyte Pub' to dance with a special person. She has Alzheimer's, or dementia, whatever you want to call it. When I first saw her, she reminded me of Beth, and still does. Beth liked to dance, and so does this special lady. Dancing with her, brings back memories of dancing with Beth, memories I wish I could relive. When the dance was over, and she left; I sat in the corner, and shed some 'fond memory tears'. Dancing with this lady helped bring Beth into the present… and it made a troubled soul smile!!

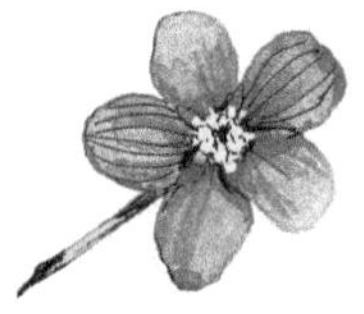

Chapter: Sad First Anniversary, without my love!

21 SEPT, 2019

It is one year since the passing of the love of a lifetime, and my soulmate, to Alzheimer's. She was, and is my everything!

I am a rational man, and I am grieving. The pain is real, sometimes all-consuming, and it sometimes feels like it will never go away. I am recovering, and learning to live life in normalcy… life does go on. I'm not trying to diminish my pain at all, nor am I trying to shame anyone into pitying me. I am trying to offer a different perspective that is helping me, and might help you deal with grief of your own… we all have some form of it for someone we have lost. Everyone deserves to recover to their former self, and achieve happiness!

And now for my 'practical', or 'rational' side, please hear me out!! After a year of grieving, along with the pain and tears, (yes, almost every day) I have come to realize that I am grieving over the fact that I still love Beth very much! I miss her presence beside me, especially on my travels (it's been my release from being home alone). I want to be with her immensely; nevertheless, none of these things will change. In essence, as with all grief, I am grieving for myself in her absence.

I know that sounds like pity, and hits the heart, realizing it may not get any easier for me for a while, nonetheless, Beth is in good hands. Think of it… she is no longer suffering the confusion and anxiety related to Alzheimer's! She is now in the hands of God, where she can walk together with Christ, and she has rejoined with the loved ones in her life that have preceded, and prepared a reunion for her! She is experiencing ultimate beauty, love, and joy, and… she is worried about my wellbeing.

On this one-year anniversary of her death, I am happy for her, and I truly wish to release her from my grief, I'll be OK! Some of the tears I shed are tears of good memories we shared, and there will be many more. Life on earth is short, and I will be with her soon; even twenty years is but a moment in history!

29 SEPT, 2019

This is not a good time for me right now, I'm still reeling from the first-year anniversary blues! I lost my soulmate, my lifeline, my anchor. I am grieving, I have a bad cold, I am in debt with my bank account overdrawn by three or four thousand dollars, I can't sleep, and tonight, I am suffering from anxiety to the point that again, I can't breathe. In the last year I have also lost my father (preceded by my mother), my aunt, and Beth's brother; all of whom I cared about deeply! Within the last five years, five of my favorite uncles, Andy, Tom, Jack, Phil, and Harvey (in reverse order of their going to the other side), twelve years ago, one of my best buddies!

As such, despondent, and ambiguous of the feelings of others; I feel I am reverting to the jerk I was before I met Beth! It bothers me deeply because I am alienating some of the friends I have left! I am truly sorry! I respect, and honour the fact that you all have stood by me, and supported me. I love you all very deeply!

1 JAN, 2020

My life is blessed, I am such a fortunate man!!!

I was blessed to find my soulmate, and the love of my life when I needed her most. She was the woman whose voice and personality I fell in love with after quitting the Air Force, and on my first day of work for Altel Data. Through what I feel is divine providence, she was available, and brought with her a son I cherish and love deeply. Life was perfect and good. We had thirty wonderful years together.

In the last seven years of our relationship, I realized my purpose in life when first, the Cancer, then the Alzheimer's took over my beloved. It was my desire to provide her care until she breathed no more. I was blessed, and it was my privilege to do so.

20 JUNE, 2020

I have been seeing a lot of a special lady lately, my lady friend with Alzheimer's. We met last year, and I am very attached to her as a companion. It is a comfortable companionship with which I give her a reason to smile in her confusion, and I gain a sense of satisfaction that I am helping this lady through her bout with Alzheimer's; much as I did with Beth. Our usual outing involves dancing at Blues on Whyte, followed with a lunch. When it's not 'Blues on Whyte Saturday', we usually just do brunch, then ride around the countryside, look at the views, and listen to music. I feel comfortable with this relationship, as I know Beth would approve; there is nothing going on; however, it doesn't mean I can't feel compassion for this lady.

Joined the Miata Club in Edmonton, and today, the date of my first club ride, I met a young lady that seemed to be new to the club as well. The familiarity of feeling out of place, as new members usually do, was a mutual feeling, as such decided to introduce myself. She is a very attractive lady, and all I could vision were the possibilities.

We formed a friendship during the ride, and yet all I could think of was cheating on my Angel with Alzheimer's. It struck me that this new relationship could never be, as how could I explain the attachment to my special friend. I felt I would be abandoning the latter for my own pleasure.

The thought of forming a serious relationship with another woman still seems foreign to me, and ridden with guilt of cheating on Beth, even if it's been a year and a half. I'm too much of a 'one woman man', my nemesis since grade 3.

14 JULY, 2020

I haven't had many dreams about Beth; this one hit my heart. In my dream, I was doing something, and from around the corner I heard Beth's voice singing. I immediately sat up in bed, and the tears flowed in a torrent! The memory of the sound of her voice was such a joy to behold. I couldn't stop crying 😢, to the point I couldn't take a breath!!

I guess my biggest fear is that I will forget the sound of her voice completely as it took a dream to bring that memory back to me. What disturbs me most is that I can easily remember the sound of the voice of almost all my friends easily; unfortunately, not Beth's, and that's what made me fall in love with her in the first place, a year before I actually met her.

God I miss my soulmate!! I know I can never replace her, and I don't want to. I'm not suicidal, and yet I would entertain the thought if there was one chance of being with her again, even for one moment. I do have faith that I will be with Beth again soon, as I know the time I have left on earth is short… based on my health, and dad's longevity, I would say twenty-three more years.

I find that as time progresses the lack of companionship is becoming unbearable!! Again, I will never replace Beth, nonetheless, during the day I find myself longing, and looking, for someone that could fill the void. There is a big void to fill!!!

5 SEPT, 2020

I have befriended a woman that has Alzheimer's, and through no fault of hers or mine, we have formed a platonic relationship, as it may be. It is a strong bond, and she cannot understand why we can't be together…in her mind, totally!! When I see her, she constantly tells me she wants to be with me, and doesn't want me to leave her!! I fully understand…unfortunately I cannot, physically, physiologically, nor financially!

She is not Beth, and could never replace Beth, even though she was, and is an amazing woman… and here comes an onset of Guilt!! It breaks my heart every time I must drop her off at the continuing care centre where she resides!

The desperation in her eyes, leaves nothing to the imagination, and again the onset of remorse!!

SECOND ANNIVERSARY

21 SEPT, 2020

Tell me all about it; you have all the answers!!! 😟

Right now, I reside between a rock and a harder place; my life seems unbearable! I am distraught on the second anniversary of Beth's death, and every familiar song I hear brings Beth back into my mind, tears to my eyes, and a full-on breakdown!! I miss her so, I want her back, and I don't want anyone else!!

In being sarcastic, even though you have said nothing, tell me again what the answer is!!!

29 SEPT, 2020

Ok everyone, it's time to come clean!!

A week or so ago, my friends were all subjected to a moment in time I'd rather forget!! On my own, I would have been ok. Sadly, I posted a lot of stupidity on Facebook, which I know worried, and offended most of them in some form or manner!! I stand sorry, and ashamed!!

As a result, I started seeing a Counselor, and though expensive, very worth it. What the Counselor said in my first session, was that I might be suffering from 'Caretaker Fatigue'; maybe 'Hangover' would be a more accurate description as mentioned in a previous chapter.

Basically, I took care of Beth for seven years, throughout the most devastating time of both our lives. When Beth passed away, not only did I lose the love of my life for forty years, I also lost a person I was taking care of full time. Combined, both losses compounded the emptiness of the hole created. As such, I was be attracted to someone needing care, and receiving care; conversely, due to my compassion, they were attracted to me. I mentioned Anne earlier in the March of 2019 timeframe, and though not the subject of this trauma, my concern for her was implicit with my phycological situation and analysis.

20 July, 2019 is when I met someone else, and the problem started! I happen to notice a lady on the dance floor of Blues on Whyte that reminded me so much of Beth in that she had Beth's sense of rhythm, and would dance to a beat much like Beth did. I had noticed her the week before, dancing with her daughter, and this week with her son. I didn't realize it at the time; however, my sister mentioned that she had Alzheimer's… I broke down immediately!!!

I felt compelled to tell her son, and later her daughter about Beth, and to offer any insight I might have gained to answer any questions they might have regarding this disease. I am not the be-all or end-all regarding Alzheimer's, nonetheless, I might be able to provide answers as to what was happening (as I am trying to do with this book).

Lack of knowledge is the big piece that was missing throughout my experience with Beth, and the angst of much of the guilt I still feel… If I only would have known things then!!! Again, I'm not a professional regarding matters of Alzheimer's, and realize my answers can only be related to my own experience with Beth; I advised them so.

Subsequently, I asked permission to dance with this dear soul, and the thought of, and the joy of dancing with Beth came rushing back. I miss Beth so!!!! Over the course of a month or so, and with a few dances under my belt, I was invited to join the family for lunch after the dance sessions and my fate was sealed.

I found joy in the companionship of this amazing woman, and it made me feel so good to see her smile… I became smitten. We became an item, even though I knew the eventual outcome, and I knew there could be no intimacy. Regardless, it made me feel so good to be in someone's life, and make them happy.

Adding to the complexities of the situation, was that I couldn't put myself out there for a normal relationship because I felt I would have betrayed the love and trust this dear lady had put in me. I was determined to see this through to the end! I again had a purpose in life! I also felt comfort with the fact that, as this relationship could not blossom to its fullest, I would have Beth's blessing, and alleviate any guilt I would feel. In retrospect, I was afraid of a normal relationship and commitment, and this filled the gaping hole in my heart quite well.

And then the hammer fell! I won't go into detail; however, concern over this relationship's progression, usurped the care being provided by the family, and they thought it best if I end the relationship. In their eyes, I was an interloper, and overtaking their responsibilities; they were right!! So, in essence, that day, I lost another person that I loved, all within two years! God help me, and in essence he has! I was getting involved where I didn't need to, and shouldn't be. I was fulfilling my requirement to keep caring for someone, and ultimately, watching her decline further, to the inevitable end, would have destroyed me. At this time, I thought rum was my only friend… it wasn't!!

Of course, there is the matter of her happiness, that some feel is unkind and cruel. I'm with you all the way, and I am now grieving for two women! I will never forget the look of forlorn in her eyes, when I left her, and it will stay with me till my dying day! It is in both of our best interests. She is being well cared for (better than I ever could), and her memory of me will soon drift off into a fleeting lost memory…as this disease does so well. When she passes, she will see that she was loved! And now, at the advice of family, friends, and a Counsellor, it's time for me to heal, and man do I need it!!

The second session with my Counselor suggested that I need to socialize with people of common interest. I used to Ski, Camp, and essentially have fun, and I haven't done that in so long. It was also suggested that I talk about Beth through my grief. Not mentioning her is not a sign of strength, and the thought of bringing Beth into the conversation with our friends would not necessarily renew the grief our friends feel. I realize they are not grieving as I do, and of course they shouldn't be, I just didn't want to open old wounds. Some of our friends might not like the suggestion, yet I need to help myself now. To our friends, my apologies. They can expect me to express my feeling, and memories of Beth freely, and more often.

In closing, I know there is no excuse for the anguish I might have caused. The actions of a depressed mind are relevant, and sometimes unconscionable!! I am truly sorry, and I love you all!!

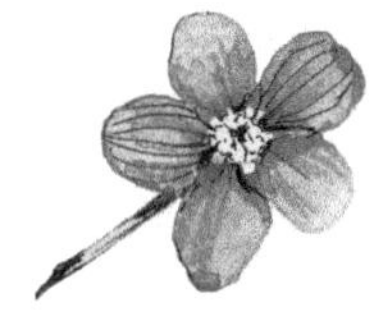

Chapter: A New Start

3 DEC, 2020 - SKIING

I've been going out into the world, and connecting with people, basically, doing what my counselor told me to do. It is nice to meet new people through the few clubs I have joined, namely the Miata Club and the Senior's Ski Club. There are so many open and accepting people, it reassures me that there is a life to be discovered out there. I've met, and made a few friends, some of them being ladies.

There is also what I deem as 'Spiritual Guidance' at play here. What am I babbling about? In a parking lot of a ski hill, on my way to hit the slope (singular, it's a small hill). I drove by a couple women, we waved and smiled at each other, and it felt nice. Skied for an hour and a half, and decided it was time to head home. In leaving I passed by these two women again, seems our arrival and departures were meant to coincide. Again, we waved and smiled; however, this time, with one of the ladies, our eyes locked as if in each other's embrace. To me it was magic!! Though she doesn't know it, my soul stirred! Nope, haven't said a single word to the lady! What occurred to me, and felt out of place was, 'why was I mentally able to accept the possibilities, without the customary guilt associated with moving on?' I realize it's early in the grieving process; nonetheless, to date the guilt of abandoning Beth has always been prevalent with every thought of connecting with another woman.

Perhaps now that I have started, and well into writing this book, Beth has deemed that this project is an important enough story, relaying a message of support and expectations regarding Alzheimer's, to release me from said guilt. Maybe I can now devote myself to finding someone, without the associated guilt; allowing me to move on. Most of you will simply think "Hogwash! It's been two tears, and you are just getting over the grief". Maybe so…or maybe not. I've made my decision; you make yours.

5 DEC, 2020

I had a bad dream during the night about Beth, and it disturbed me greatly. We were driving a dark blue rented vehicle, and we were stuck in a snowbank with a couple other vehicles. I got out of the vehicle, with Beth behind the wheel, we were able to push her off the snowbank. As she drove away, I panicked because neither Beth or I knew where we were; she had Alzheimer's, we were in a strange city, and she took off on her own.

I hopped into my vehicle (don't know why we had two), and tried to catch her. There were a couple cars between us, when I had to stop for a light, Beth drove on, and I lost sight of her. I turned down a few streets trying to get a glimpse of her; nonetheless, it was hopeless!

This represents the worst-case scenario you could ever experience, the loss of a person under your care, with no way to find her. I woke up with an anxiety attack, I couldn't breathe, I was sobbing, I was heartbroken, and there was no hope!! In my waking moments, I told Beth, "Why are you doing this to me? I can't take it!! Don't do this to me ever again!!!!"

I needed my sister's guidance with her innate ability to decipher dreams to make sense of it, which she did very well!! Her translation was that 'Beth driving away with no hope of finding her' was indicative of her leaving me, and would not be returning; it was over! Sounds bad, yet not so!

There was more to the dream, which also fell into place. I went into a restaurant to finding the Manager, I passed a fellow at a table that was challenged in some way, and had just been served a plate of chicken. The fellow then dropped his food on the floor. Uncharacteristic of my usual self, I didn't stop and help him pick it up. This was deciphered as me being released from the shackles of caregiving for someone incapable of caring for themselves; indicative of what my counselor said to do to allow me to move on with my life.

Sometimes it's important to change, and face a new challenge as we progress on this blue marble around the sun. When you finish taking care of someone (which eventually happens), regardless of how close you are to them, you must realize you've done all that you've needed to do, and can do no more. Life does continue, and you must become part of it without them or lose yourself in the dust.

7 DEC, 2020

Wishes do come true!! God granted me a special Birthday wish last night! ☺

Well, tonight I dreamt of Beth again. This time we were on top of a building somewhere; seemed like Spain for some reason. I could see pigeons eating on a couple roofs off to the distance, and below my level. Beth had just returned from somewhere, and things were fine; we discussed her trip for a good period of time, yet, with no specifics. I then thought of, and told her I missed her, and was happy to have her with me again. That's when I thought of Beth's Obituary as George printed in his paper. He published a poem, and the words that came to mind in my dream were:

"If I could have just one more wish,
And wishes did come true,
I would wish to have one more day with you!
I'd tell you of all you've missed… … ."
That poem always breaks me up inside!!

These weren't the actual words of the poem; nevertheless, that's what came to mind in my dream. Anyways, I thought of the poem, and realized that Beth was visiting me; the obituary wish was actually being fulfilled. I was able to tell her how much I missed her, and understood she would be leaving soon; tears of joy filled my eyes, and that's when I woke up!!!!! I was so happy!! 😊

So, thank you God for the only present I've ever needed since Beth's passing, 'to have one more day with you'!!! 😭😭😭

9 DEC, 2020

In March of 2019 I recounted a story about Anne from the Westlock Continuing Care Centre. As an update, her deterioration came quickly; she requested, and was accepted for the MAID Initiative, and underwent the procedure on 9th December, 2020…Gilles' birthdate. Again, I have lost a dear friend, yet relieved in the thought that she is no longer suffering, and has reunited with her soulmate, Gilles. Here's to you, my friends!!

9 JAN, 2021

Well, it happened, after I told Beth to never do that again! Obviously, I'm missing the point. So, what happened? Had another nightmare about losing Beth!

I woke up at 4:00 a.m. or so, after my usual banana, and about an hour on the computer checking emails, I went back to bed. Woke up at 6:30 a.m., in distress, and in a panic situation. I had lost Beth again, same concept, she had Alzheimer's, and we were in a strange City… Chicago, I think. This time, we had just finished a conference, and were packing up to leave our hotel room, suddenly, Beth was gone.

Of course, that's where panic set in. You cannot imagine the trauma when suddenly, the one you are mindful of, and tasked to take care of, disappears. The search started immediately! I went through the rooms, then the hallways, and carried on into the rest of the hotel; conference room, restaurant, kitchen, lobby, then eventually outside. That's when the real desperation sets in; which way do you go, what do you do, who do you call? It is all so hopeless!

I then head out in search of the most precious person in my life, with apprehension, and knowledge that she can't find her way back. I hastened down alleys and streets, I looked in different buildings, I explained the situation, and ask everyone I met if they had seen her; the realization set in that I didn't know what she was wearing. I went into a business which had a beauty parlour as a front with a restaurant/bar attached as part of the back of the building, again asking if they had seen Beth.

Left and went to a nondescript office building. That's when another challenge hit me… I had lost my cellphone in the process. My thoughts were that it would be impossible to find because it was a desirable phone, and would have been kept by the finder, especially in a strange city, so it was worth the backtracking. Neither the restaurant/bar nor beauty parlour had seen it. Headed back to the hotel and the conference room. The people I was in the conference with lined up, and said they would help find her; they only looked in the conference room.

Then I went to another building, where someone got me to follow them to an elevator, and left me there. There were two men in the elevator. They were talking and laughing, nothing related to Beth; regardless, I chastised them for being jovial when I was in distress, looking for my wife that was lost, and had Alzheimer's… not funny at all.

Then off to the next building, with an exterior elevator that went up the building diagonally. Two young kids had joined me, and when we got to the top, which was at ground level, it was like getting off a flatbed truck. There were a couple big snow lumps about two feet in diameter that we had to kick off the truck bed to get off.

Back to the restaurant/bar, still no cellphone, still no Beth! I noticed I was walking as if I was drunk, and under extreme fatigue, for some reason that disturbed me. I guess the thought was that no one was taking me seriously. Headed back towards the hotel… all hope gone; no hope left!

That's pretty much when I woke up. I had an intense level of anxiety; however, what bothers me most is the amount of guilt I felt. I could understand if I had neglected Beth in her need, or even if Beth had died in an accident that was my fault, nonetheless, why so much guilt??? I did everything I could, with the knowledge I had, during her care; why is there so much guilt haunting me? I wonder if this is a common occurrence with someone that has lost the love of their life, perhaps survivor's guilt?

I realize the symbolism of the dream in that, with Beth's passing, she is lost to me, and I will never find her on this earth; however, why do I still try to find her when there is no hope of doing so, awake or in my dreams? I do know my journey is not yet complete, even though things are getting better. Regardless, if these nightmares of losing Beth persist, I will be seeking additional help from my Counsellor.

25 JUNE, 2021

It's now been almost three years since Beth's passing, and I feel I must continue the saga.

So, at what time does the grief of losing the one person in your life that means more to you than life itself, do you transition the grief of not having that person with you at every turn of your life, to the thought that you are just plain lonely? When does missing someone, become missing anyone? When can you accept that you need some form of socialization without feeling guilty that the social time is not spent with your soulmate? When do you accept the fact that she will never return, and it is OK to seek the fulfillment of love, without the guilt of it not being the one you lost?

What it boils down to are the choices available to you. You can continue the path of loneliness, existing without, but in constant reflection of, the perfect life you had; or start from scratch, and struggle with trying to forget the constant comparisons you make with every new person you meet, and accept the possibilities; they are endless, and that is what scares you. It's like being an awkward teenager again; however, not with the expectations of what the imagination must create, with the knowledge of what perfection is. You're not excited with anticipation; you're terrified with fear of the disappointment of regression with the potential of rejection. At 74, the last thing you need to do is tell someone that it's not working out… and the loneliness continues.

10 JULY 2021

The story goes on, but what does recurringly come to mind is having lost my soulmate. Right now, I'm impossible to love! Think of it, someone might be attracted to me, and the possibilities are endless; however, I have lived the life of attaining a soulmate, and unless I fall in love with the demeanour and personality of someone before even meeting her, recurrent of how I met Beth, how can I love her back? It would be unfair for me to lead someone on with the potential of them falling in love with me, still with the expectations that she will not measure up to my expectations. I know it sounds chauvinistic and egotistical; nonetheless, think about her. How do I let things progress, if I don't feel there is serious potential for being a soulmate? Leading her on, for my sole pleasure and gratification, is the definition of being chauvinistic.

I have met two potential suitors, neither of them will talk to me, and rightfully so… I am definitely 'out of their league'. Again, I desire a soulmate, and as the term reverberates continually in my musings, perhaps it's time to embellish my thoughts of what a soulmate is. Next chapter…

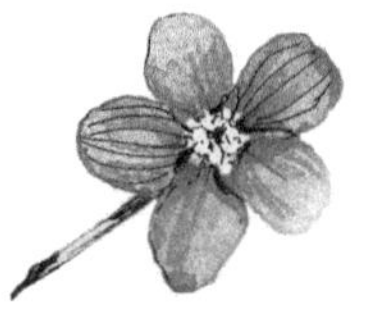

Chapter: Soulmates

I mentioned 'soulmates' often in this book; so, what is a soulmate?

They say, "Opposites Attract". That may be true; however, it is just that, an attraction! Those relationships rarely work out. Think of it, why are you attracted to a person of opposites? It's probably just the thought of intrigue in seeing a change in your life; the desire to conform the person to your will; or maybe because you admire the person's attitude, intelligence, or even their dominance, and that's just to name a few off the top of my head; mostly attributes you don't see in yourself. Problem is, for that relationship to work means either they will have to change to become a mirror image of yourself, or you will have to change to match the qualities you admire of that person. Not an easy task. Don't get me wrong, sometimes it works out.

Conversely, meeting your 'Reflection' may have its issues as well! Can you really live with yourself for the rest of your life…or theirs? To be attracted to your double, you really must love yourself, and be totally self-absorbed and happy with that concept… forever! Ah, boredom comes to mind! Boredom, of course, will propagate wandering of thoughts, interests, and probably disfunction as an inevitable solution…this can be applied to extra marital sexual relationships. Problem lies in the fact that your partner will, or maybe not, have the same tendencies, and their desire for change may not align with yours.

So, what is a soulmate? My definition is two people who are compatible, selfless, have common intelligence, and common interests; that can suggest, and accept new ideas and thoughts; be able, and willing, to admit they were wrong, in conjunction with being able to forgive and forget; and most importantly, be able to respect each other as equals. It's not about belonging to you; it's about belonging with you!

Beth and I had this in Spades!!!

DO SOULMATES LAST FOREVER?

For the most part yes, and yet not necessarily. How could they? Fundamentally, when you stop being equals, the relationship is over! There are so many factors to be considered though, time, and the world, are constantly changing. So do people!

I talked about 'Opposites', and about 'Reflections of Yourself'. What if a person transforms into one, or the other, which happens all the time? There are psychological, and/or medical issues, that can change a person's perception of life, sometimes to a point that becomes unbearable for the other. There are physical issues that can interlope on one's own personality in ways detrimental to a mutually agreeable type of relationship. A person might become disfigured, or handicapped, and you might love the person regardless of the physical aspects, yet more difficult, personality changes as a result. There is drug and alcohol issues, which have a propensity to change a person.

And then, there are mental issues that can occur. Of course, this falls in the medical category, and is relevant to my situation. Beth developed Alzheimer's through no fault of her own. I had the choice to abandon her because she was changing mentally; however, as she regressed, and became a different person, my love for her only grew stronger. It's all part of growing old together, we all deteriorate, some in different ways, and at different rate than others.

So, when do you pull the plug on a soulmate relationship? That's totally up to you, how much you love your spouse, and are willing to accept living in the unimaginable. Many of the above factors can be self-propagated, and some can, or can't, be avoidable. Leaving a true soulmate will probably never happen...you're all in, thick or thin, and yet, living in an unacceptable situation should never be forceful or guilt ridden. No one should be blamed for abandoning such a relationship. Shit happens!!

LOSS!

Now that I have imparted my definition of a soulmate, you cannot imagine the concept of losing your life partner, your soulmate, unless you've experienced it. Can you imagine knowing seven years ahead of time, that you were going to lose her? Not suddenly, as in 'she will die suddenly in a car accident then, so we still have seven years of continued zest and enjoyment of a normal life together', instead, in seven years of gradual deterioration, not of body but of mind, the essence of what makes ourselves 'us', and our bond unbreakable!!!!

First, and immediate thought, is that you must provide the ultimate care, provide acceptance, understanding, and capture and cherish every moment available, so as to reinforce the love you share with her...until the end. Gradually, her love fades, emotions wain, and life itself drains from the essence of the person she was. Now live with that going forward.

I'm struggling with life right now! I loved going on rides in the country with Beth. We both loved the serenity and seclusion of the outdoors, something an urban lifestyle can't afford. We loved driving around, picking up rocks, for no other reason than their beauty. I specifically enjoyed admiring, and photographing the beauty of a sunset; the desperate attempts of a deserted barn to exist; the random patterns of the branches on a deciduous tree with a haze subduing the light of a background Sun during the winter months.

We enjoyed parking the car facing the sun during a cool winter day, and feel the warmth it provided us as we rested with our eyes closed...perhaps even catch a few winks of shuteye. These were the things that meant something to me, especially with Beth at my side. Now, nothing seems to matter anymore! How can I have such a love of God's Nature, and a distain for life? It's easy, when you have no one to share it with!

I desperately want to regain what I had with Beth, yet how can I? She passed away, and I'm left with a dilemma. I think of, and feel the desire for a new relationship to renew and experience the love and joy of my former life; however, all I need is to have Beth's memory reappear, and I'm a basket case. It would be so nice to be able to talk to someone again! I don't need conversations for the sake of making and hearing sounds, I need to be able to have a meaningful conversation, and dialogues that creates memories, such as those that Beth and I were able to share. I want to love again!!

So, how do you replace a soulmate? The answer obviously is… "You can't"! Do you realize how hard it is to find one? It can happen, yet what are the chances of finding another soulmate, and would you want to? There is a peculiar dilemma you are faced with… are you trying to find another soulmate for yourself, or are you trying to be a soulmate for someone else? Soulmates are the ideal relationships; the product of mutual interests and respect, evolving over time, and cannot be established based on past experiences. Once you've had that experience, it seems nothing short of that will suffice, and you'll never attain that form of relationship if you try to 'replace' the one you had with a new one; it must come naturally. Quite a quandary!!

CAPTURE THE MOMENT!

Communication is one of the things I miss the most with the loss of my soulmate. We used to sit for hours, with a beer in hand, and talk of plans, wants, issues, or whatever else came up. It's ironic that, as they say, sound is the last thing to go when a person is dying, and yet, unfortunately, conversations was one of the first things to go with Beth. I went through five years of sheer agony! She would say lots, yet I couldn't understand most of it. There was a lot of "Yes Dear!" "Unh Huh!", and "is that right?"

I know it sounds like I was placating and demeaning her, except it wasn't that at all. The other choice was to ask her to repeat everything, or tell her "I don't understand", or even worse, "What the Hell are you talking about?" When a person feels frustrated in not being able to be understood, and reminded of that all the time, they will eventually shut it down. The one thing I didn't want is for her to stop talking altogether! It was frustrating for me; nonetheless, necessary for me to hear her voice.

I was able to make out, the three words that would melt my heart occasionally, "I Love You!" One of the last things I recall her saying was, "I'm so Lucky!" Those words will remain firmly intrenched in my mind forever!!! It not only reaffirmed that what I was doing was appreciated, it meant that she understood she was having unsurmountable difficulties, and that I was doing the best I could. It also signified that she knew I loved her, and I would always be there for her.

This brings me to my discussion point, and perhaps some valued suggestions. In our time of grief, we remember the special conversations, or exchange of words that occurred under special circumstances. What we don't remember, with much regret, are the everyday conversations, where the sound of her voice captivated the soul. I so wish I could remember conversations and inflections imparted during supper, or even watching TV. These are the instances in time that are non-conscience occurrences. Things that occur in your life in the blink of an eye, or the beat of a heart. Take this advice while you still have your soulmate with you, make it a point to consciously remember some of these uneventful conversations and moments. After the fact, I wish I would have made it a practice of doing so. There is so little I can remember.

On a relative note, there is ample documentation available on the Internet, regarding losing the memory of the sound of a loved one's voice after their death. This is very disturbing to discover after their passing! In this day and age, it is so easy to record, or even video your loved one having a conversation during an everyday event. What a treasure to have and behold! I have some videos, though there are not many, that I will guard with my life. I have some of Beth in her declining years; however, the few I have pre-Alzheimer's are priceless! Get out that iPhone, and hit record, NOW!!!

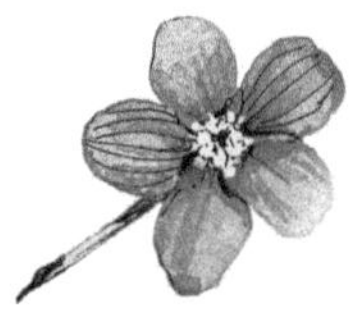

Chapter: The Elephant in the Room!

I would be remiss if I didn't address the Elephant in the Room… that being suicide. Now please bear in mind that this book is based solely on my experience respective to Beth's release from Alzheimer's.

Before I delve into the crux of the matter of suicide, and recount personal experiences pertinent to my situation, I feel I must provide a bit of psychology relating to humanity in general; it is important. To understand suicide, and its potential as a consideration, I must reiterate that this book is written from a male perspective as there is a difference.

As stated, before fifty, the woman's natural tendency is to be the caregiver for the family. When the family transitions into being 'empty nesters', the tendency is to continue caring, be it for grandchildren, ailing parents, or a spouse in need, or they lose their sense of purpose.

After fifty, a woman will continue to be a caregiver, within an extended family dynamic, or society as a whole, becoming a wise, and revered shaman (or in modern terms, an elder). If that family dynamic fails to present itself, a woman tends to relinquish her requirements to be a caregiver, and will embrace her newfound freedom to find a diversion. As such, a woman will then establish a new identity, outside of her family dynamics, and expand her horizons into artisanship or entrepreneurship; her purpose in life doesn't seem as diminished.

Men, on the other hand, feel the need to provide and protect family until the provisions of life are taken care of. In prehistoric times, they taught a male child the role of hunter-gatherer; in modern times, to amass wealth, property, and possessions. In either case, when prosperity has been accomplished, they can then retire from their role as the father figure, and desires to drink beer, and watch football (just kidding). A male has completed his initial identity, and now wants to be more involved with the family, and their care, yet the family unit has been disbanded, relatively speaking, and he has no one to care for except an independent spouse.

Essentially, their roles have reversed.

Fundamentally, before fifty, the woman's focus is taking care of the family. Man, on the other hand, upon retirement, reverts to nesting, and growing old with their spouse. Take either thing from those respective roles, and they lose their purpose in life; in their psychological psyche, there is nothing left to live for.

Again, this book is written from a male perspective; however, is relevant to both genders. The trauma experienced by the female gender will be nothing less, yet the outcome could be vastly different.

The loss of a loved one manifests itself in many ways! My life changed from the familiarity of happily living with my soulmate, to the trauma of watching her deteriorate over a period of seven years, and then, losing her to the afterlife. That's when my life transitioned into a life of grief with depression of a love lost; the forlorn loneliness of living an empty life without her by my side.

As you are well aware by now, I've reiterated a plethora of overwhelming emotions I experienced. Now that I've lost my soulmate, I contemplate what others might be going through. There is a fine line you walk while feeling the disparage in the loss of your sole reason for living, and the overwhelming grief and desperation you are faced with; I fully understand how that could have some considering suicide.

The potential is very real, very serious, and not to be taken lightly. I've had a personal exposure to this potential, in the suicide of my aunt Cecile, just before the imminent death of her husband in palliative care, suffering from throat cancer. They had no children, and it was more than she could bear. I understand her plight, and I miss them both very much.

Another example of the overwhelming grief that can ensue, is regarding Pablo Picasso, who died on 8 April 1973 from pulmonary edema and heart failure while he, and his wife Jacqueline, entertained friends for dinner. Devastated and lonely after the death of Picasso, Jacqueline could no longer justify her existence, and killed herself by gunshot in 1986, when she was fifty-nine years old.[3]

I in no way mean to trivialize your grief at this juncture! Her death is, or will be, traumatic and horrific. I was fraught with guilt of being released from the burden of caring for her; I did all I could, and yet, it didn't seem to be enough! I understand what you are going through. These are strong emotions that overwhelm the mind and soul; the very fabric of your being. The path laid out before you may, at times, seem very bleak and worthless; nevertheless, survivable.

I am by no means a professional on this subject matter, and I strongly suggest you seek professional help in dealing with these emotions. My only intent in bringing up this devastation, is to reflect what I experienced, and perhaps prepare you for what's to come.

Have faith my friends, you are not alone! Many have traveled the path of being forlorn and lonely, a path you foresee ahead of you. Again, don't hesitate to reach out for help and support from family and friends; most importantly, from the professionals of the world.

---

3 *Kimmelman, Michael (28 April 1996). "Picasso's Family Album". The New York Times. Retrieved 26 August 2010.*

CONSEQUENCES

It is important to consider the consequences of your potential actions, specifically suicide. The following consequences referred to, are written to help you cope, and perhaps realize that the anguish is not yours alone, and not your sole burden of responsibility.

After I lost my one true love, my soulmate, I often thought I would welcome ridding myself of this mortal Albatross. At times, I find there is really nothing to live for, and would welcome my demise with ecstatic pleasure.

There is always the possibility of catching Covid… maybe that's God's way of providing me with an out… or maybe, it's God's way of isolating me, and giving me time to write this book… see all that God does for you?? There is always the possibility of contracting a terminal disease, although the likelihood is slim; my dad lived to ninety-six, and was healthy as an OX, he just faded away, I have twenty-two years to go… "Oh boy!!"

Now you may think I'm still skirting the issue of 'Suicide', but no!! It's easy to 'check out', as there are many possibilities to end it all; however, there are far too many consequential factors to be considered. My dad taught me to always think of the consequences of a deliberate action.

What comes to mind is driving in the path of an oncoming vehicle; that could be swift and final. Although, who is in that other vehicle? A service person on his way to his retirement function? Newlyweds? A graduate of Medicine that is on their way to saving countless lives? A newly born child? Perhaps one could drive in front of a Semi… that wouldn't harm anyone, right? Unless one would glance off, and hit another vehicle with the same consequences as mentioned above; or maybe the car would explode, and take the life of someone that was trying to save your life, maybe even the driver of the Semi!

OTHER CONSEQUENCES

What I am feeling, with my loss, is very powerful, and all consuming! Grief, depression, and guilt, are emotions you as well must contend with; It's not easy!! The thought of a life of grief and loneliness is not something that any one of us are looking for. Yes, the thought of ending it all enters my mind, and I feel forlorn, as I'm sure you will or are as well.

Yes, you lost your soulmate, and are having great difficulty surviving without her; nonetheless, you also must consider the feelings of others. As bad as you are grieving, there are probably several people that, while grieving for the same person as you are, will now also have to deal with the grief, disbelief, and anger, at the loss they would now feel over you. Your circle of friends has been important to the both of you, as part of your social group for some time, and have now become part of your support group. Take time to reflect on the situation, and you will discover that, conversely, you feel empathy for your friends as well. They are closer to the situation than you may think, and they are there for you as you for them. Mutual support is what helps guide us through the grief! It's all part of life, and they are part of it with you!

I personally would never consider suicide for many reasons. Firstly, for me it's not an honourable way out! I was in the Armed Forces for ten years, and though I never faced imminent danger, the thought, and possibility of death was always prominent, and training was such that there was honour in sacrificing life and limb for your country and fellow man.

Unfortunately, the same cannot be said for some of our serving heroes; the ones in the military that have faced the enemy; those Police Officers that have witnessed trauma in the streets; the First Responders that have lost a patient regardless of the efforts afforded them; those that are now facing PTSD! All too often suicide seems like their only recourse. I understand their anguish, and I wish them well! God be with you, and thank you for your selfless service for my freedom and safety!

Second reason I have for suicide not being a consideration is that morally, with respect to Christianity, renders it unacceptable. Now you can claim, rant, and rave about the non-existence of life after death, and/or the existence of heaven and hell all you want, irrespective of your thoughts, I don't give a shit! After all, what makes you, or I, or anyone for that matter, the expert on anything regarding life, death, or anything in between, before, or after. You, as I, are nothing except a spec in time, a burden on the environment. Why we are here is not for you, or any scientist to decide or even try to explain. That being said, I've seen far too much evidence of life after death to feel I need to deny the existence of God and the afterlife.

In summation, EVERYONE will experience what you are feeling at some point, you're not the only one going through this!!

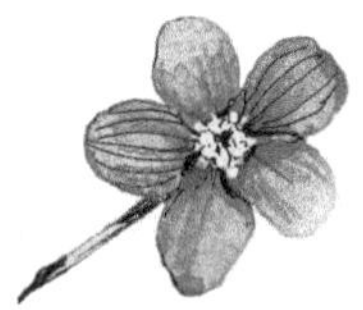

Chapter: The Downside!

EVOLUTION OF GRIEF!

"A heart that's broke, is a heart that's been loved!"[4]

Perhaps 'Evolution of Grief' is a bit of a misnomer. Not sure what stage of Alzheimer's your significant other is at; however, my experience has spanned seven years, and then three years in absentia. What I found, is that my fear and anxiety were prevalent in the earlier years, morphing into grief as time progressed, and her responsiveness regressed. I was losing the one I was familiar with, the one I was comfortable with, the one I loved deeply, one day at a time. I thought I was prepared for the grief, and that most of the grieving would be over…not in the slightest! I've lived the five stages of grief many times over during her decline; once she passed away, the full-on grief took place!

So then, what is 'Grief'? Focusing on the loss of Beth, grief is the loss of life itself. My purpose for living, and the life I once knew, were gone; forty years of my life was suddenly whipped out…all that was left were the

4 Ed Sheeran from the song, "Supermarket Flowers"!

memories! In her absence, it feels like a part of me was ripped out of my body; not my heart because I still, and will always, love her; not my brain because I continually go back to her treasured memories; no, more like my stomach because there is a big hole left in me, and the hunger and cravings cannot be fulfilled! Not nearly as romantic; nevertheless, more depictive of the true feeling.

Grief is not a 'one size fits all', nor is dealing with grief! Every life is different, every loss is different, and everyone's perspective of such is different. The loss of a child, a parent, a sibling, a relative, a spousal partner, a friend, a pet, even a celebrity can perpetuate grief of varying degrees. The loss can be tragic, or a blessing in varying degrees, and everyone will experience varying degrees of their own grief for the same loss! What I'm trying to emphasize is that it is impossible to cover every aspect of every loss for everyone.

On earth, we are subject to all sorts of suffering, from the time we are born till the time we die. Suffering can be both physical and psychological. It goes without saying, that physical suffering is never easy to endure, or watch; however, there are medications to control pain…to the point of comatose.

Our experiences with the animal kingdom predicate that we euthanize animals in these dire situations; we haven't gotten to that level yet regarding our human counterparts…almost (the MAID program option). With a prognosis of improbable recoverability, under a Personal Directive, we do authorize removing a person from life support, and that makes common sense.

Psychological suffering is a completely different ball of yarn!! Unlike physical suffering, in this situation the person is usually, but not necessarily, unaware of their disability, and there is no recourse for cessation of life; nor should there be!! What I'm referring to covers all forms of psychological duress; Psychosis, Schizophrenia, Bipolarism, etc., etc., etc. In these situations, people can lead normal and productive lives, as there are medications to stabilize the condition until they pass away from otherwise natural causes. Not so for Alzheimer's, the regression is slow, constant, and terminal!!!

In a perfect world, we would divest ourselves from the anguish of grief, in that the person we cared for, the one that was suffering either physical or psychological pain, was not suffering any longer. In essence, their pain is over, and whether you believe in the afterlife or not, they have been freed of their constraints. We should be comforted in this outcome!

'Nuff said… so why the grief? It's simple! It's because it is about the pain YOU are feeling, the absence of a familiar life and lifestyle YOU have lost, and the loss of the companionship YOU have grown to appreciate. It is all about YOU, and there's nothing wrong with that!!!

When you lose someone dear to you, time has no relevancy, and the grieving imparts upon you a sense of hopelessness, with the perception that it will last for an eternity… or at least till your own demise. What it all boils down to, is that life is only yours for a temporary blip in time with which grief will drag on and on to the end… if you let it. Hopefully you realize that you are becoming ineffective as a human being, and need to readjust your priorities; some fail to realize this, and opt for the unthinkable!!

There is no easy recipe for you to overcome your loss. You feel outrage, pity, remorse, and sometimes guilt at the thought of the suffering to which your loved one was subjected to. You also feel grief in how the loss impacts you.

All I can speak of is my own personal perspective with any form of validity. I saw my beloved deteriorate from the vibrant, intelligent, funny, and loving person she was to the end. I took care of her for seven years, of which the last year and a half, were in a continuing care facility as it became impossible for me to manage her on my own. It was the best attention she could possibly get! Even then, I was with her almost every day, from the time she woke, till she went to sleep. My only reprieve was that for one day a week, I was able to visit my aging father at his continuing care centre; point being I was only away from my soulmate for four hours of that day.

My wife passed away on Sept 21, 2018; her brother unexpectedly, from complications of Alzheimer's as well, on the 11 Nov, 2018; my father, at ninety-six years, on April 22, 2019 (Easter Monday); and a dear aunt (dad's sister), on the 11th of May, 2019… the day after the internment of my father. It was a bad year for me. With all this in mind, your grief is no less trivial than mine!

In my particular situation, a very deep love of my wife remains. What I miss the most is her presence, the conversation, the feeling you get when you hug one another, and of course the intimacy. I will always feel a lot of love for Beth, and in her absence, I miss every one of those interactions very much. Nonetheless, if I cannot be comforted in the thought that Beth is in a better place, with assurance of our gradual reunion, then life has no meaning for me! It's sort of like, "Absence makes the Heart Grow Fonder" with one exception…the absence will never go away until I die, and we are reunited. That is why the grieving persists.

Now to my point! With Alzheimer's, you, as caregiver, are subjected to the feeling of desperation, as you see your loved one deteriorate into infancy; a seven yearlong agony for me. As I said previously, I thought most of the grieving would be over. I thought I would just grieve her deterioration until she passed away, and then be relieved that she would be in a better place, at peace, and with clarity of mind; that would be it… yeah, as I am discovering, not that easily dismissed!

Now, a different type of reason for grieving took over! What I had not considered is that, although I grieved during her seven-year deterioration, the life of love, joy, and fulfillment that was prevalent, prior to her dementia, came back tenfold. That was one aspect of grieving I wasn't prepared for while she was still with me… a double whammy!!! Now, with the three years after her passing, and with proper counselling, the grief and guilt has subsided somewhat. While driving, the hole in the stomach is still there when I hear a sad song, and she's not there beside me; yet I can function.

We are social beings, and as Covid has pointed out, there is so much sorrow associated with not being able to hug, or even being allowed to visit family and friends. With the heartbreak and grief of not being able to see, or even hold your newborn grandchild in your arms for over a year. More specifically, not being there to hug, hold hands, or being present to show support to those that we have lost.

God bless social media and Facebook; nonetheless, it pales in comparison to the real-life experience of unity through closeness of being. I cannot imagine, for one moment, the angst of the horrific situation of standing by, and losing someone within close proximity, and yet out of your reach during their last moments on Earth. I was so fortunate to be able to be with Beth during her deterioration of mind and body to the last moment. God took pity on me, and I feel very blessed and grateful to not have to have been separated from Beth at the end. My heart goes out to all of you that have suffered a loss under Covid conditions.

There are many that understand your pain and grief, because we all go through some form of it. Additionally, it disturbs me that there seems to be so many people grieving with no hope for closure. My only optimism is to bring some form of understanding, some comfort, some hope, and some faith to you, and everyone else that is suffering.

Grief is a normal part of life, and given time, should subside; if not, seek out professional help. It doesn't have to morph into a tragic loss of yourself, with no chance of recovery.

PERSONALIZING GRIEF

In saying that, grieving is purely personal! You are grieving for the person you lost, nonetheless, they are gone, and there is nothing you can do to change that; in grieving, you wish you could.

If you could replace the void created by the loss, you would no longer grieve, you would simply relish the memories. That's the trouble, too many people simply try to replace a loved one, and it rarely works out. The replacement will never be the same, and that's what you so desperately want.

You must allow yourself to feel the pain of the void. Eventually, you find other distractions that allow you to evolve into the new you. Then, and only then, can you honestly commit to someone that has their own personality and traits to which you are attracted. Some traits may be the same as your previous partner, and that's OK.

New relationships can be successful because you do bring to the table the experience learned from your previous relationship. You've learned what works and what doesn't, what you like and what you don't, what to look for and what to avoid! In essence, your past relationship will continue, and that is beneficial to a budding partnership.

New relationships with someone that has also lost a partner is interesting, and quite common as you have a mutual mindset. Part of that relationship must be that you, and your new partner, must be allowed to digress, and share in the memories of your past relationships. That's what life and love was built on! To not be allowed to remember and share, will create a sense of guilt of omission that will fester to the death of your new relationship. You cannot just stop remembering, and quit loving people from your past! That was, is, and always will be part of your life! When will I stop grieving over Beth? When I don't love her anymore!!

Now, there is a caveat regarding a new relationship that you must consider!!! You don't want to share 'in' each other's grief, what you want to do is be able to console each other when either of you go through a bout of grief. You must understand the emotions they are going through, be it to provide empathy, a distraction, crying together, or leaving them to isolate till they work through the pain. You don't want to both be continually living in each other's pit of pity.

This also applies to how you are handling your grief as compared to the grief of someone you are in a relationship with. They may not be as emotionally connected to someone you lost. As an example, this could include losing your parent, sibling, or one of your close friends. Of course, your partner will also be grieving, yet it may not be to the extent that you are. With grief, if you overly obsess you risk losing your partner as well simply because they can't assimilate your level of grief. They will get over it much more quickly than you will.

I know that sounds harsh and cruel; nevertheless, realize that no amount of grief will help or be of any benefit to someone once they have died. You need to lose the obsession of grieving over the one you lost, and change your focus to the ones around you that matter most, or you could lose them as well…a double tragedy! You will still grieve, and should be allowed to grieve; however, it must eventually become 'on a personal' basis, and acceptable to your partner.

Of course, none of this applies to the loss of a son or daughter, especially at a very young age. I cannot imagine the grief associated to that situation. That level of grief has at times been so overwhelming that it has caused the separation of many loving couples. Something you must consider when trying to find a new partner. Will they, or you, depending on which partner has suffered the loss, be able to withstand the immense grief? It's something that might never end, and empathy can only survive so long before it alienates the union. No one is at fault, it's just what happens. You must place yourself in the other's situation… either way.

GUILT

I use the word 'Guilt' a lot in this book, and it bothers me. The thought that you will feel guilty because of words I have written can be an overwhelming imposition on your wellbeing, and what you are going through… you may not feel any guilt at all, and that would be OK!!!

When I use the word 'Guilt', I want to assure you that I did nothing wrong! I don't feel guilty for something I have done; I feel guilty in wondering if I could have done something better. If I could of, in some way, eased her anxiety, confusion, and discomfort.

That's but one form of guilt! Another is guilt associated with the thought of cheating on my wife; that guilt is surreal!! It was unconscionable while she was alive, and yet that is what is hardest to rationalize. I fully realize she would want me to move on; I realize there is no way she would judge me as cheating on her; I realize it's irrational to even feel I am cheating; nevertheless, while we were together there was no need to have some of these feelings, and now they are forefront in my mind. After three years, I'm still cheating!!!

According to 'Psychology Today', "Guilt is aversive, and like shame, embarrassment, or pride, has been described as a self-conscious emotion, involving reflection on oneself. People may feel guilt for a variety of reasons including acts they have committed (or think that they committed), a failure to do something they should have done, or thoughts that they think are morally wrong."[5]

Prior to her death, I felt what seemed like guilt to me, in that I saw my soulmate deteriorating before my eyes, and the natural instinct to protect the

5 Psychologytoday.com/Guilt

one you love was foremost in my mind, yet there was nothing I could do. The cure I wanted to provide was unattainable! The word 'Guilt' may be the wrong word to use at this time, and yet the thought festers and is relentless.

Realize that guilt is something that is synonymous with grief! Grief is a feeling of remorse after the loss of someone you loved; guilt is the thought that perhaps you could have, should have, would have done something different while they were still with you. As such, grief is predominantly felt after losing your spouse, of which, the guilt is for thinking of not doing everything you could have before her death. Even 'Survivor's Guilt' can predominate, and the perception that it 'should have been you' is overwhelming.

Guilt; however, goes back a lot further! Relating to your spouse, every wrong you've ever done, everything you failed to do, every time you lost control comes back with a vengeance exponentially, when you are grieving. Have faith that you are not alone, and do seek professional help.

Guilt also manifests itself in other ways as you move on! I so crave the interaction I enjoyed with Beth for thirty-nine years, and my mind wanders towards being able to share that companionship with someone, almost anyone; again, along with that comes the guilt! I have so much love inside to give, and yet I don't want to give it to anyone but Beth!

The thoughts of holding someone in an embrace is a powerful need that I've enjoyed and shared with my loved one for many, many years. Now, when I think of Beth's embrace, I relive the memories of what I had, and break out in tears. When I think of embracing someone else, I wither in guilt! It is a dilemma! The thought that she is in heaven, watching over me with sadness and shame, or perhaps with love and approval… who knows what is right or who is right?

To reaffirm my situation, my wife was diagnosed with Alzheimer's seven years prior to her death, and I was by her side from the onset, almost every day from the time she woke till she went to sleep. One of the last things that I understood her saying, about six months before she passed away was, "I'm so lucky!" So powerful, and yet, I still feel guilty in that maybe I could have done more before it was too late; maybe even before she was diagnosed;

maybe she wanted to travel more, or she wanted something that I didn't provide, or even that I should have danced with her more before diagnosis!!!

In the last year, when she spoke, she was obviously trying to say something; that, in of itself, was imminently important to me. I have a video of Beth just prior to her death when she tries to say something to me; I watch it, and it breaks my heart. It is repeatedly horrifying to me; she says something, and I can't understand her last words!!! The torture she must have been going through to try to figure out what she needed to say, then not being able to formulate the words, must have been devastating. The grief is in not understanding her last words; the guilt is in not being able to understand what she was trying to say.

I'll assure you of one thing, after watching her lie in her bed, and able to do absolutely nothing except breathe for eleven days, makes me wonder why she had to go through with that experience at all…or me for that matter. It would have been so much more acceptable to ease her of her suffering as soon as she could no longer swallow food or water. That is when there was no longer any hope for revival. That was it, just wait for her to pass away!!!

Those eleven days of my life I will cherish, and will haunt me forever!! The lack of certainty of what I could, or should have done, is thwarting my peace of mind. In retrospect, I wish I would have just swabbed her mouth with a wet sponge more often, even just brushed her hair; I was so stupid!!! Maybe the guilt stems from me wanting to be there to ease her transition to the other side in some way, to comfort her while I watch her take her last breath; a moment I regret missing.

LONELINESS

Ah, the one thing you never think about until it grips you, and you feel you need to do something about it.

So, at what time does the grief of losing the one person in your life that meant more to you than life itself? When do you transition the grief of not having that person with you at every turn of your life, to the thought that you are just plain lonely? When does missing someone, become missing anyone?

I need to address this topic because it is integral with death itself, and yet, more poignant with Alzheimer's; something no one touches on. After seven years of caring for the one you love, and then three years of the never ceasing heartache which forebodes your need to socialize (breaking down in public is never fun), you become lonely, and crave companionship. You not only lost the one that you loved and cared for deeply, you also lost the one that cared about you; most significantly, loved you.

Even Counselors don't get the point! The advice is to "go out there, join a social club, socialize with a group of normal people, not necessarily with a support group of grievers, and not someone in need of your care; just get out there!!!!" The preceding quote was not actually suggested verbatim, and I fully admit to taking creative license on my interpretation of what was suggested at the time. Regardless, after thirty-nine years of marriage, the last seven of which were spent focused on the care of my soulmate, and being seventy-four years old, for me, getting out there seems akin to stepping out in front of a Bus.

You can't hold, hug, or kiss a memory; nevertheless, you can share it…but with whom?

Yes, you have friends, and at first you feel it would be so nice to move in with them, to be able to recount the memories, and relive the relationship you've enjoyed in the past; the things that made you friends. You know it can never happen, and never will. Besides, you don't want to impose on them, and have them be encompassed in your pit of pity. They were friends with your spouse as well, and at one time grieved, and were sorry for their loss; nonetheless, that card can only be played for so long. Subsequently, you see them in ever decreasing occasions, and even though you grieve on, you know they have come to terms with the loss of a special friend.

You could move in with your children, you know they would be more than welcoming… for a while. Eventually you become part of the furniture or worse, the babysitter if they have small children, or even worse again, 'the handyman'. Don't get me wrong, they would appreciate having you around to take care of them as you did for the first eighteen years of their lives. I mean hey, they are now taking care of you… "oh excuse me, I have to go unplug the toilet, while I'm there I can stop the water running after the toilet is finished flushing… change out the toilet for a new one… no problem!"

I do get tasked with maintenance and reno duties from time to time, and I enjoy the distraction from wallowing within myself. I am fortunate to see my family once a week, and thoroughly enjoy my time with them; it's sad that some families are geographically separated, disallowing them to reunite more than once a year or so. Nevertheless, I could never be subject to living under someone else's rules, especially at my age… now I know how they felt for those first eighteen years.

I know this sounds ridiculous; however, the point is… are you ready for this… it does nothing for your loneliness! The loneliness grows with time, and you may think to yourself that three years is bearable. What no one realizes, is that because your partner was deteriorating physically and mentally, you were gradually been socially secluded. You didn't feel lonely at the time, because you were preoccupied with the one you wanted to be with and cared for deeply. Then, it all ended! There you were, two steps in front of the bus I mentioned earlier.

And the Guilt!! Again, I continually revert in hindsight to the Guilt!! It is now three years since Beth passed away, and it just seems so inappropriate to even socialize without sharing that experience with your wife; you were a team! Conversely, while she's still so vivid in your memory, the feeling of shame in even thinking of cheating on your wife with someone else, all becomes overwhelming.

So, what is an appropriate passage of time, and from when does it start? Three years? Seven years? Ten years??? The latter has been the term of my celibacy, and yet, I can't get over the shame of simply thinking about companionship, much less intimacy. I want to get on the bus; unfortunately, it's travelling at sixty miles an hour, and I just got my legs in motion. Don't know whether to keep walking, step aside, or just stand there.

Alas, I will get over it! Everyone does… if they need to.

RECUPERATION

So, what is the distinction between when you are simply replacing the love in your life, or finding a new life filled with love? I have yet to find a middle point, a time when I can cherish the memories of the past, and find comfort in the action of the new. You might feel okay having a meaningful conversation, and eventually, hugging someone, nonetheless when will you feel comfort in the intimacy?

At what stage do you capitulate to the guilt of thinking you need some form of socialization without your soulmate being that source? At what point is the guilt superseded by the need? When do you accept the fact that she will never return, and it is OK to seek the fulfillment of love without the guilt of it not being the one you lost? You do have to move on with your life eventually; when, and how…and the loneliness continues.

What it boils down to are the choices available to you. You can continue the path of the loneliness of existing without, yet in constant reflection of the perfect life you had, or start from scratch, and struggle with trying to forget the constant comparisons you make with every new person you meet and accept the possibilities. They are endless, and that is what scares you. It's like being an awkward teenager again, yet not with the expectations of what the imagination must create, but with the knowledge of what perfection is. You're not excited with anticipation; you're terrified with fear of the disappointment of regression with the potential of rejecting, or being rejected. At seventy-four, the last thing you need to do, is tell someone that it's not working out.

There is, however, a fine line between the distinction of loneliness, and simply just missing your soulmate. After three years of grieving the one I lost, I have come to realize that it seems I am no longer lonely and am just missing my Beth. I seem to be quite OK with being alone. The need for companionship has waned; and yet I will always miss the companionship of my love lost. Maybe that's when recuperation sets in and a person gives up on any thought of replacing a loved one, for the thought of starting anew.

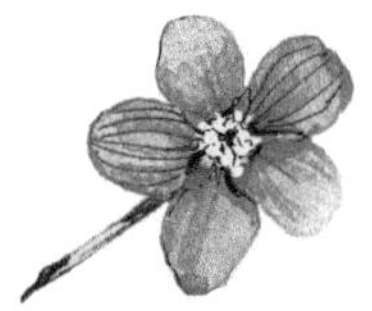

Chapter: Finding Solace

Before I go any further, I must emphasize this disclaimer. I feel that every one of you will have issues with the following, nevertheless, that is not my intention whatsoever! The following is solely my perception of care relating to my personal experience.

I understand that this disease manifests itself differently, and the experiences of every patient, friend, family member, and caregiver will be different. I in no way mean to trivialize what you are currently, and/or have been going through. Please read to the end, and understand that I have a great deal of empathy for each of you. If I can give even one of you a little bit of solace, then it will be worth it.

In the preceding pages of this book, my reasoning has been that with every disease, other than Alzheimer's, there is a ray of hope. Many have a potential for a cure, or some form of control, that allows the Patient to lead an extended and productive life! With Alzheimer's, there is no hope, no cure, and certain death as the outcome! I felt that with all the fundraising done for these diseases, with relatively little going toward Alzheimer's, that if simply one year of fundraising of one of those diseases could be diverted towards

Alzheimer's, a cure could be found. My reasoning could not have been more flawed, and I sincerely apologize to every one of you!

I met with a good friend of mine a while back that totally changed my attitude, and put things in perspective. Her husband passed away after a long and painful bout with cancer. My dear friend was a nurse, and she said, "If I ever catch a terminal disease, I hope it's Alzheimer's". I was stunned as this caught me off guard! I asked why she felt that way, and she responded, "Of all the diseases, it's the only one where you simply, and relatively painlessly just fall asleep!" It made me question the rationale behind finding a cure for Alzheimer's! Potentially, if they do find a cure, they might save millions of people, only to have them die a horrific and painful death from some other disease or accident. Of course, that is flawed thinking on my behalf because there would be far more patients, and their respective caregivers, that would lead normal and productive lives with their spouses, allowing them to actually 'grow old together'…something I no longer have the privilege of doing.

That's when I realized that it's all about me!! With the agony of witnessing the gradual decline in Beth's functional, and mental capabilities, it was I that felt the agony! The thought of great memories of the past, were my memories that could no longer be share with her anymore! The loss of recollection of whom I was, was all about her forgetting me! The constant requirement to feed Beth every meal, was all about my feeling sorry that it had to be done at all! Furthermore, the distress of not knowing if she had soiled herself, and needed cleaning, was my distress! The feelings and emotions that I experienced, were solely my own.

Don't get me wrong, it is a long and arduous disease to live through and care for; however, if you can remove yourself from the mental anguish you are feeling, it is much more bearable. You will definitely feel the trauma; nonetheless, be at ease that it is only you experiencing that trauma. By segregating your distress, you are not being callous about what the patient is going through, you are being realistic about what they are experiencing. Truly not much different than caring for a newborn, except in a reverse order. You don't get to revel in each new ability learned, instead, you feel distressed at each nuance of life lost. Feel good in that what you are doing is your best, and what needs to be done to ease her anxiety. If there's one thing I did right, it was to try to always be there with Beth during her waking moments.

I firmly believe that, with Alzheimer's, God has allowed hearing to be the last sense to go for a reason. It's a proven fact that music is the one thing that can temporarily bring a patient back from the void during the final stages. There are a couple movies that I highly recommend regarding this phenomenon; one called 'Of mind and Music', and the other 'Alive Inside'. In being with Beth through this tumultuous time, my voice and music were always there to give her reassurance, strength, and comfort in her unending state of confusion. That is what an Alzheimer's patient needs the most!

I wish I could reciprocally have heard, and understood her reassurance, strength, and comfort during her unending state of confusion; that's what I needed most!!!

MOVING ON

A few things are coming into play here that few people are aware of yet may help. I mention many times that I don't want to replace Beth and I would like to recapture the life I experienced with Beth. It now occurs to me that in feeling the need to move on to find companionship, and perhaps even a lasting relationship, I keep looking for the same qualities I found in Beth; why fix something that isn't broke… oh yeah… it is broke!!

What I overlook, is the possibility of finding someone with different qualities that would provide me with a totally new perspective on life. Not as much 'different than Beth's' qualities, more so attributed to being a different person. That way I could remember and relish the memories of Beth, and not have to compare those to my newfound relationship. It would add to the qualities I so enjoyed with Beth, leading me to enjoy an ever-growing expanse of experiences in my life. New experiences that would mould me into a new me. Somehow, it perhaps will alleviate my guilt because I am not finding a replacement for Beth even though I still love her so!!!

To explain, when you found your soulmate, your spouse, your lover, your life changed. Perhaps it was out of duty that you got together due to an unfortunate sexual encounter, and your morality commanded that you step up to the plate… Kudos to you, my friend! Perhaps it was out of desperation that you felt the need to conform to the norms of society, and become part of a union which has endured to this day. Perhaps, like myself, you found a soulmate for whatever reason.

I'm not trying to vilify anything in finding a soulmate; I'm trying to establish a point, and here it is! Your relationship obviously flourished to become true love, regardless of the reason for your union, or else you would not be reading this book. Point being, that as that relationship grew, you were transformed into the loving and caring person you are. I'm sure many of you will attest to the fact that your significant other did in fact become your soulmate.

In being your soulmate, or even a significant other, you found something in that person that you wanted to share. In my advanced years of twenty-nine, I simply found Beth's personality traits, and her demeanour, so desirable while dispatching 'Techies' to a trouble, I wanted to spend my life with her even before I met her… 'until death do us part!!', and I would have been happy to continue that lifestyle to my end.

I can only speak for myself because I have experienced the ultimate tragedy in the loss of a soulmate; whereas, perhaps you are just beginning on this journey. I want to express that there is hope for your enjoyment of life going forward.

Two years after my loss, I found myself trying to find Beth's personality traits in someone else, so as to continue with life as though nothing had changed. You know that can't happen, and the wrong concept to carry on with! Don't get me wrong, it could happen, and I'm happy for you if it does; however, don't discount an opportunity to delve, with pleasure, into a new reality that will transform you yet again. With one more year under my belt, I am encouraged.

There are countless people out there that will be stuck with the same dilemma you will be faced with in trying to replace someone. That, in of itself, is locking them into the thought of not being able to regain the existence they once had. Open your heart to new possibilities, new experiences, a new love you could flourish in, and with! It's not about forgetting your lost loved one, it's about sharing the great memories, and friendships you have shared in the past, with a new perspective going forward.

I'm not suggesting you should change, not in the slightest. Just be open to new possibilities. One of the things I enjoyed most with Beth was going for drives in the country to experience nature at its best. Perhaps your new squeeze has never been out of the city during her life, taking her for a ride might be new, enjoyable, and maybe even overwhelmingly beautiful for her. Conversely, you might be a Country Music fan, and she is passionate about Opera. Let yourself experience something out of your norm, you might be enthralled… if not, it may not be the right relationship for you.

Best advice I can give is go slow, take it easy, try the old, experience the new, then make a decision.

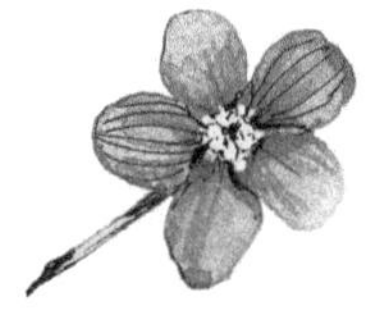

Chapter: Spirituality

I DO BELIEVE

Throughout this book, you will recollect that I expound in the belief of a Higher Being. What you believe in, or what I write for that matter, is irrelevant in the care of your loved one. My belief comes from the many experiences in my life where the unusual, unexplainable, or even simple coincidences, have occurred; too many to not believe. My interpretations of these events are personal, meaningful, and pertinent to my situation in life. As such, I no longer feel the need to deny God's existence by my silence. I find comfort in his presence, and I have been blessed far beyond my worth.

My intention is not to make this book a religious statement, as you might think. I made references to God many times; it was how I survived! My intention is solely in that perhaps you can find solace in the unrelenting task ahead of you. Spirituality predominated many of my thoughts while caring for Beth through Alzheimer's which is what this book is about. If that offends you because you're an Atheist, too bad!! I do not intend on sounding derogatory, all I mean is that as a non-believer, in your hour of need, you can't find comfort in God, as I did. By the way, ever think that maybe God doesn't believe in Atheists?? If you deny the existence of God, or any other deity, what are your options, a six-foot hole in the ground? God times zero equals zero! You got nothing Buddy!

Humm, I should write a book "Fun with Atheists!"

LIFE AFTER DEATH.

Of course, I would be remiss again if I didn't explore the post dying process. I watched a documentary in which a Buddhist Monk was asked what he thought the experience of dying would be like; the response was both enlightening and surprising. He said he would compare it to having an orgasm… interesting concept from a Celibate Monk.

So, what does happen after she passes away? There are two perspectives on the topic: Life After Death – 'the Science' and 'the Spiritual'! The science is irrefutable to some. The spiritual; either you believe in the hereafter or you don't, and I will never change your mind.

With that in mind, as this book reflected my experiences with Alzheimer's, and my wife's death, I will focus on my perspective on this subject, and on the thought process you might go through after your loved one passes away.

What I need to transpose to you is there are two aspects to your psyche; what goes on in your head? The first thing that will hit you, is the onset of the grieving process, something you will, and must go through. Of course, this pertains to you, and for each of you this will be very personal, specific, and different.

Second part of your psyche is, what happens to her after dying? More so the 'OK, she has passed away, now what?' aspect! Thoughts of the afterlife, whether you believe or not, will bounce around in your head, wondering if, or hoping there is a hereafter, and will you be able to reunite with your soulmate. It is a nice and comforting thought!

THE OTHER SIDE

So, let me enlighten you! As I said, the science is irrefutable in that the person is cremated or is buried, and the decomposition starts; either way the outcome is dust. Spiritually is a bit more complex and controversial, and yet a little less defined. If you don't believe in the hereafter, then the conversation is over… Good night! If you do believe, or are interested in a bit of Socratesial questioning, with a smattering of humour, read on!

We think about life after death, let's talk about life before birth. Do you remember anything??? Thought not (except for those few that have been reincarnated of course)!

Why is it we were born innocent and leave guilty? We're all guilty of something…except maybe Christ, Mother Theresa, and Princess Dianna. It's the time in between that is the issue. Everything we know, everything we've been taught, every belief we have, has been learned; some for the good, some for the bad. Once we cross over Jordan and enter the hereafter, are we then responsible and accountable for our actions while here on earth?

I guess the point I'm trying to make is we are influenced to believe whatever we have been taught; is a Dictator any more responsible for his actions than a Saint? We are the product of influence.

To counteract my point, which must be done to assess any situation, we are born with a free will; it is our choice on which action to take, good or bad. Guidelines are provided by religion on morality, and by the government on laws to follow, some choose to not follow same, or are taught to rebel against these teachings. As an example, what if you are influenced to think that killing an infidel is just and right…death is irrelevant? Are you judged as evil, if you think you are doing the right thing?

So, what's it like on the other side? Heaven? Nothing? Everything? All the beauty of earth…and more? What if heaven is simply just another step to 'Nirvana' or 'Valhalla'…or the other way around? How about hell? Is there such a place? What is the final judgment that gets you into hell? The minimum requirement? Is there a 'Get out of Hell Free Card?' If God loves man, and heaven is nothing except love, why would God create hell for some to suffer? If I go to hell for swearing, do I get punished the same as a child molester? Yeah, for some there must be a hell!!

Christ told us that if we followed his teachings, we would attain heaven, what he didn't tell us, is what heaven is or is like? 'The house of my heavenly father' doesn't explain much. What do you think?? Streets paved in gold?

Why? I would just as soon have a dirt path through the woods. Do you get a mansion? Is that what it's all about, or even wanted? Interesting questions.

What about people that suffer through the pains and challenges of mental issues all their life, like a person with Down's Syndrome, Autism, OCD, Scrupulosity (a subsets of OCD surrounding a discrepancy in their religious or moral beliefs). Perhaps they suffered through other diseases like Crones, MS, Cancer, Alzheimer's, or even Alcoholism? Do they attain a better place in heaven than I do because they were inflicted and suffered on earth through no fault of their own? God knows they deserve it; at least I believe so! I've led a charmed life on earth, maybe this is my heaven, and as good as it gets. In reality, I could not want for more, and as such do I deserve less in heaven?

What if someone cheated you out of $100.00? Will they be indebted to you in heaven? In this world, where justice presides, would it not be fitting that they would owe you in heaven? Yet, what is $100.00 worth in heaven? What if they go to heaven, and you don't? Do they still owe you? Worse outcome would be that they went to hell, simply because they owed you $100. Maybe the lesson to be learned, is to forgive, and love everyone while here of earth, can you truly do that right now? Heck, it's only $100.

Will we meet our loved ones again? How about the ones we didn't particularly like? The ones we truly disliked? What if 'they' were more righteous than 'you'? Will you still dislike them? Will you have to bow to them? Maybe serve them? Are there any labour camps in heaven?

What about your soulmate? Will your earthly soulmate find someone better in heaven? Stands to reason that there is always someone better. Will you even meet up in heaven? Maybe they will reside solely with family, and never the twain shall meet. Maybe the heavens will be so full of love, that you will love everyone there equally, and there is no such thing as loving your soulmate more than anyone else. Will you be united with them again for eternity… as you now desire?

So many questions, so little time…and so much to consider! Is it any wonder people are afraid to die? And yet, those that have had an 'out-of-body' experience usually come back embracing death, or at least not being afraid of it. Was their experience actually passing through the 'Pearly Gates' or just peeking inside? I could just go on forever!!

People never think of the possibilities when faced with limitations, yet we all dream! We dream of winning a lottery, nevertheless, the possibility is so remote some don't by a ticket. You may not believe that the fork ran away with the spoon, or that the cow jumped over the moon, or even that pigs can fly; however, if you don't buy a ticket to a lottery, you will never win. I can say or make fun of anything that you don't believe in, and you should not get offended. If you don't believe in a Supreme Deity, or the existence of an afterlife, then what I say should be of no consequence to you. However, think of the possibilities!

If there are no earthly bounds to cause you pain and suffering, if your body, with all its functions and limitations ceases to exist, if you no longer feel the confusion and anguish associated with Alzheimer's, the possibilities are endless. After all, why were we born on earth with all these limitations, only to have it all end with no chance of reprieve. The fork will never run away with the spoon, the cow will probably not jump over the moon… (why would she want to?), and why wouldn't pigs be able to fly? Will you win a lottery? Each and every day for eternity! Will you be able to reunite with the one you saw disintegrate into nothing? It is a must!

The Yin and Yang of life must prevail! The suffering and sadness you endured, in the care of someone so special, needs to have a Yin (or Yang). The confusion and anxiety your loved one endured, has to be rewarded with clarity and ease of mind, and the desire she will have to express her gratitude for you, which she could no longer do, will be played out; it cannot simply end as it has… unless you still don't believe… pity!!

KARMA IS A BITCH

We all know the saying that "Karma is a Bitch"! Karma is when you're driving along, and you catch up to someone going 10 Kms/hr. below the limit. That '10 Kms/hr. slower' gets to you, and a clearance finally opens up, so you put the pedal to the metal, zoom past, and "Wham", 56Kms/hr. over the limit, and a court appearance. Yep… true story!! The Karma part is when the dodler drives slowly by, feeling sorry for you… yeah, right!! We've all been there!

Karma only occurs maybe once every thousand times, and it seems never for you. The ones that bite you are the worst. Such is the way an Alzheimer's Extended Health Care Specialist can expect 100% of the time. Every time they lose control, lose their patience, or the patient feels even the slightest hint of aggression, or frustration, they will express anxiety towards the Health Care Specialists, and they will remember it for quite a while. The care provider becomes the face of anger, whenever the patient sees them. As a caregiver, it is important to hang bad emotions at the door.

Imagine; however, as being the 24/7 caregiver of your spouse, you have no door to hang your emotions on as you're already inside. If you want to survive this journey, you must totally divest yourself of these types of emotions while with your loved one or face the wrath of Karma, not a pleasant situation!

The alternative is a blessing you can enjoy. Replacing frustration, anxiety, and hopelessness, with patience, understanding, and love, does make you a much better person. You also get to reap the benefits of becoming a calmer person, and having peace, harmony, and requited love in what's left of your relationship. Caregiving will not become a profession; it could; nonetheless, become a job you can enjoy.

As a caregiver, take it easy on yourself, and do what you must do without expectation of affirmation. Leave your emotions of anxiety, distain, grief, and guilt behind; life will be so much easier on you if you do. There will be ample time to reflect, and you will be plagued with those uncharted emotions long after the loss.

ANGEL'S ANGELS!

Angels are sent to us in our time of need! They protect us from harm; they direct us to make the right choices for our preservation (you don't know why you hesitated, or you turned left instead of heading right, as you normally would have); they come to us when we are distraught, and need guidance; they comfort us when we are alone and lonely; they even perform miracles on our behalf when the end, or our downfall, is imminent, and there is no way out… unless you are an Atheist of course!! (Just kidding! Even atheists get angels, although they are non-appreciative of such).

In many ways we have been blessed by 'Spiritual Guidance'… it happens to all of us at some point in our lives! Once we have been consoled, guided, or saved, we are thankful for a moment, then go on our merry way. I firmly believe that Beth has been my guardian angel many times in the last couple years. I have what I consider as 'doubtless' evidence; however, the recount of such would render the pages of this document quite lengthy; perhaps fodder for another book.

There are other angels amongst us. Not just the ones with wings and halos 😇; the ones we see all the time! I'm talking about the human variety. The ones that give selflessly to help and comfort others, with minimal, or no compensation, or recognition. Sure, some get paid, as it is their livelihood, and heaven forbid, they do have to eat sometimes. Some just do it out of the compassion of their heart as volunteers, and they continue to do it with no end in sight, simply because we need the assistance.

In a hospital environment, we have nurses and aids that perform all that is required to assist in the care and comfort of the patients. This group are elite, in that they do all they are trained to do, and so much more. Sometimes they work under severe distress, brought on by a patient in their care that did not understand what was needed, or why. Regardless, they carry on, and do it day after day after day!!! When my dear Beth was with us, I saw this time and again. The care they provided, where I was not able to, went above and beyond any expectation of human compassion and kindness! They are truly angels as well!

What people may not realize, is that in a continuing care facility, these angles will continually take care of the same patient, from the time they are placed in their care, until the patient dies. This could take years, and within that time, unbeknownst to the patient's family, bonds are formed. When a patient succumbs to the ravages of their infliction, there is an impact on these health care specialists as well; they then continue to work without the grieving process they need so much!

These angles endure unspeakable stress in caring for our loved ones for years on end, and then help to comfort them in their final hours!! They are simply amazing heroes that deserve the most gratitude that can be afforded the best of our country's elite! They deserve a Military 'Medal of Honour' for dedicating their lives to the protection of others.

Now to my point!! If you will notice, there is a common denominator, 'it is about **YOU**!' Not in the sense of your ego or desire for attention, moreover, in the sense that these angles look out for you, fulfill your need to ensure your loved one is cared for, and it seems to be a 'One Way Street'!!!

What happens when angels need help? Who will be their angel?? Who, looks into their lives, and says, "Let me help you"? Maybe they need you to simply talk to them as a friend from time to time. In many ways I feel this applies to both our spiritual guardians, and our human ones.

It may be a little harder to provide help for our spiritual angels; nonetheless, maybe they need confirmation of their help with more gratitude than "Thanks, see you next time I need help!" Maybe they need a prayer as recognition, or perhaps even just assurance that we will change our ways to prevent our needy requirements! Maybe they need to see that we'll eat healthier, or stop smoking, or drive slower, or as the ultimate 'Thank You', we will in turn help others through our experience.

It pains me to think of the human angels amongst us that, after doing heroic deeds during the day, simply go on their merry way, or go home, and deal with the frustration, distress, hardship, pain, and loneliness in their lives by themselves! Know this, that as I needed your help and love, I will be there for each and every one of the healthcare nurses and attendants in any way I can in their hour of need.

Thanks for all that you do, and for your support provided me to help me continue with the rest of my life. 🙏💗

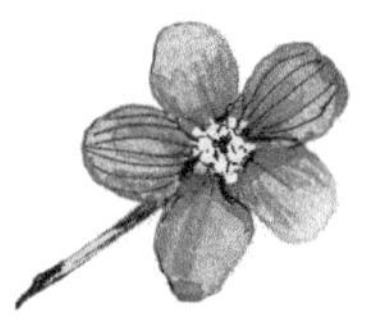

Chapter:

I'm ready!!

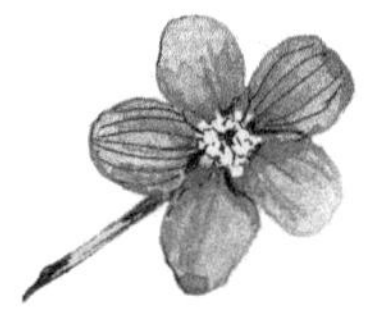

Chapter: Oh Well!!

Well, that was short lived! I thought I was ready for the next chapter in my life!! Well, not so fast. It seems things aren't over till they are over.

This is an addition to the book that will not be reviewed by anyone; these are my words, and my thoughts! It's the life I am, and will be subjected to live from now on… and it ain't pretty!

Warning: *What you are about to read contains graphic thoughts that some readers may find disturbing. Reader discretion is advised.*

I stand before you a dejection of a man… so lonely, so missing the one thing I need, Beth! This is the point where people think of the unthinkable. Why is there no reconciliation? Why is there no comfort? Why am I still here?

Now that my life has returned to the miserable existence I lived before finding Beth, I now wonder what was it worth? I lived the perfect life for thirty-nine years, including the time my love disintegrated into non-existence; now, nothing!! There is nothing left!!

I put myself out there, and thought for a moment there was reprieve, but no one could come close to Beth. It's not that I'm not willing to look at a new life; it's not that I don't feel the urges to commit to a relationship; it's not even that I don't try; it's just that nothing comes close.

I met someone that could move me… two, actually. One didn't return my call, and the other wants me for my chainsaw. Here's a sample of the texts:

Her: - "Hey, if you're free tomorrow afternoon, would you like to come to a garden party? My back yard, party for two ppl. I've been working on the garden, but I need a break."

Sounds pretty enticing; even romantic! Is this my time to reconnect with life? My chance to find a recourse to this emptiness overtaking my life? That text was followed by…

"Also, if you'd like to bring your chainsaw… I have one branch by the garage my cousin forgot to cut it. Thanks!

It was a great BBQ, followed by watching a rousing game of hockey, watching the Oilers loose, and then… Good night! See you soon.

Don't get me wrong, she is a fine and beautiful lady; one that anyone would like to connect with… and we will remain good friends.

So back to where does that leave me? I have a feeling that this chapter in my life is far from being over, far from being resolved, far from becoming what I had, and back to my awkward teenage youth, with many unfulfilled years to come!

What was it all worth??

As time passes you sit there, and think of those that preceded you. You lose part of your life one acquaintance at a time, one friend at a time, one relative at a time. Then, you lose the one you loved the most, the one you relied on most, the one you cherished most, the one you can't live without. That was your life, and it has culminated into nothing. You miss the ones you cherished, the ones you hated to love, and the ones you loved to hate; mostly, the ones you loved to love. They are all part of the life you treasured, the life you were comfortable with, and the life you had; then you realize, that's the problem; the life you had with these special people can never be experience again.

"Time to move on!", they say. Time to get a new life, find new adventures, new loves… but how, what, and with whom? Do they not realize you can't find new relatives? Do they not realize how hard it is to form new and everlasting friends with common interests? Do they not realize how hard it is to find a new soulmate from scratch when you're seventy-four?

New adventures? Do they not realize how hard it is to even do something different, and out of your realm of enjoyment? Give up camping, dirt biking, and take up crib card playing? That's an extreme, perhaps; however, even trying to like golf, or bowling, when it's not your 'thing', is not a change you want to even try. Helping others is a chore; volunteering is a chore; caring is a chore… when you're seventy-four.

New life? What's left for you; perhaps only twenty more years of memories, twenty more years of missing the ones you loved, twenty more years of loneliness, twenty more years of trying to rebuild your life? Any, and every, time you try to get back into your former life, you are brought back to reality with sore joints, muscle aches and pains, disappointment in the loss of capabilities, and stamina. You're old, and getting older. Life must change; you must change; you don't want to change! Only twenty more years of misery… you're only seventy-four! What is it all worth it?

You no longer have any ambition to leave the house. You no longer want to clean the house that you don't want to leave; don't want to cook; don't feel like doing the dishes. You find you no longer want to make the bed… heck, you no longer want to get out of bed! Is it any wonder people change to become despondent, and depression sets in? Your 'Bucket list' turns into a 'Fuck-it list'! You can no longer live the life you had; you can no longer have the life you lived? Is it any wonder people gravitate to a life of substance abuse? Is it any wonder people commit suicide? No, I'm not suicidal; nevertheless, I understand why some are. Is it all worth it?

You were all hoping for a happy ending… so was I! Sorry to disappoint you, there can be no happy ending with Alzheimer's. The trauma of watching the one you love slowly disintegrate and die while you watch, while trying to help, is a mountain too hard to climb, and yet once you do, there's another mountain in front of you! Those last few words spoken that I could understand Beth saying, "I'm so lucky!" reverberate in my heart. Was it all worth it? Then yes, now… ? That my friends, is grief!!!

What you have just read constitutes a serious bout of depression. I did not feel this way yesterday, and I did not feel this way in the following days. If you have, or find yourself experiencing the same emotions I have just expressed, there is a very high probability that you have the same depression and desperation that I felt. It seems overwhelming and hopeless! If you are experiencing these feelings on a continual basis, you must seek professional help!

Many, in fact all people, that have been traumatized, either through caring for an Alzheimer's patient, or even experiencing the loss of a dear pet, go through the same desperation. There is no shame in grieving, and feeling lonely and lost, there is no shame in sharing those feelings, and there is no shame in seeking help. You can get through this, and rise above the grief; it will never go away, but it is survivable.

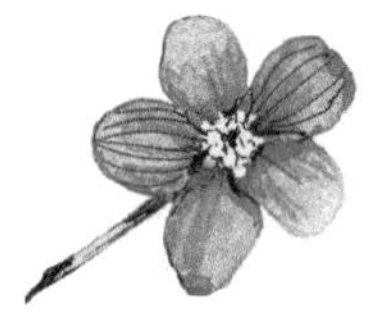

Chapter: Reflections

While editing this manuscript, there were a few reflections that came to mind on how I could have handled things differently regarding Beth's care, and yet were not forefront in my mind at that moment in time. I felt I needed to expand on those thoughts for information, clarity, and to perhaps help you react differently when encountering those incidences.

Although some of these reflections may not relate fully to my caregiving of Beth, I felt were pertinent to me and might help establish my persona, which is a large part of this book. It is hard to understand the emotions if there is no connection to the sensitivity.

RETROSPECT… IN LOOKING BACK

The passing of my mother on 23 Sept, 2012 was mentioned almost as a side-line of Beth's care. I feel I must regale a bit of history regarding my parents as they were integral in my upbringing and help set up the foundation of my respect for, and the love of Beth as a soulmate, and why I was so dedicated in her care.

I mention my dad many times in the annals of this book, as you are aware, not out of disrespect for my mom, simply because my mother passed away during the early stages of Beth's Alzheimer's journey, which is the focus of this book. It does behoove me to provide a little background regarding my parents, the background of my existence.

My parents were the product of farming, pioneering stock; strong willed, compassionate, dedicated to the nurturing of family, and the need to survive through unimaginable hardship. A love that endured and flourished for seventy years, then beyond my mother's death, to that of my father's. They were both strong willed, and that strength of character propagated times where they were at loggerheads with each other; never violent, and never with disrespect… just difference of opinion.

My mother was a very strong woman and underwent such emotional angst most, in today's society, cannot fathom. It is traumatic to lose a child at birth with a grief that some see as unsurmountable; my mother lost two girls before I was born, then another girl between my sister and I, then two more girls after my second sister came to be. This is a trauma that, for a young boy at the time, I did not perceive. I now live in wonder, respect, and admiration of her, and now that I fully understand, I cannot imagine how she was able to function, and still provide the parentship I was subject to. Love and miss you mom!!

Although it seems I never appreciated my mother as I should have, I always had respect for her. The one thing she taught me, that I take away from our relationship, was the utmost respect for all of womankind. Nevertheless, being the only male child, and the first to survive, I was always the apple of my dad's eye, and treated as speciality over my sisters; yet again, to both, I'm sorry! I'm sure I will be beholden to the ladies of my family when we meet beyond the Pearly Gates. Don't get me wrong, I don't feel I was spoiled… well, maybe a little; nonetheless, I felt the sting of the strap as much as my sisters.

Many in today's society will expound the horror of such abuse; however, I always deserved my punishment, and it formed within me a character of respect for others that is so lacking in today's wimpy, non-respectful, 'ME-ME-ME' society. I thank my parents for the discipline, and the love I received. It has served me well!

NUMBER TWO

Beth and I were loyally involved with the Rimbey Lion's Club, and it was a large part of our lives. It was a necessary trauma inflicted on me, when we had to quit as members of the Lions Club on November 28th, 2013. If you recollect, at the time Beth became reserved, and felt uncomfortable in social surroundings. As time progresses, this will impact your life as well, and something to think about in advance. If the Rimbey Lions Club would have been aware of Beth's situation, it would not have been as traumatic for me, as to quit without a forgone purpose. Though resigning was not an imposition for Beth, following are reflections on how involved we were, and how much I had to give-up.

For those unaware, the Lions Club is a non-profit organization that raises funds in support of the local community. I have never met such a pleasant group of committed individuals, that use this purpose to make gatherings so much fun. There were many times we were selected to perform in parts of skits during one of our biggest fund-raising events, 'Pancake Day', in Rimbey.

I've had to sing to Beth on stage, with a less than perfect rendition of Satchmo Armstrong's 'What a Wonderful World', while both of us were dressed as clowns; dress as a Beauty Queen, even though cross dressing is not my thing…not that there is anything wrong with that; appear as a baby in a diapers, reminiscent of 'Baby Huey' (now I'm dating myself); Muckluck Charlie dancing the Can-Can while supporting snowshoes; and in a three-year-old version of a famous sports champion…with my booming voice, I was the Curling legend, Hector Gervais (if you can imagine me as a baby, following my mom around, hollering, "Sweep!…Sweep!… Hard!").

During the Rimbey Lions Club 60th Anniversary, we played multiple parts in a flashback of entertainment stemming from the encompassing sixty years. The production lasted three hours where I played Lou Abbott in 'Who's on First', Eddie in the show 'Greased Lightning', etc., etc., etc.

Many times, I've been put to task to dress as a wine induced clown (a cross between Clem Kadiddlehopper and Freddie the Freeloader comes to mind) to entertain members, visitors, and guests; a part I fit naturally into… I've had a lot of practice.

And now, looking back from the present day (April 2021) some of you might be thinking that, as Beth and I made so many friends with the Lions Club, that perhaps I should get involved and rejoin the Lions again, however, I couldn't! All the good memories were with Beth, and she wouldn't be there.

Getting together with such a dynamic, fun group of people is what everyone dreams of, I just can't get my heart into it! It would be like becoming King… of lower Slobovlea! It seems funny, there are so many things I enjoyed doing when Beth was with me, even when she wasn't an active participant, in which I have absolutely no interest in doing now; photography, camping, country drives, sitting around a campfire with a cool one in my hands… nothing seems to drive my ambition anymore. Covid isolation seems a blessing; I guess that's how grieving works.

ONE MORE

Back in September, 2015, while reviewing thoughts of the current situation, she wanted me to teach here how to use tools so she could be an active participant in building some projects; I commented that it was an impossibility as she cannot grasp instructions at all.

In retrospect, I now wish I would have tried to teach her. Power tools would have been out of the question, yet I could have given her a hammer and held the nail for her to pound on (better my fingernail than hers, and I would gladly do it now). I put more importance in completing a project and I missed a golden opportunity to share the valued time with her that I now wish I could recapture. Any opportunity to do things with her would now be treasured to elation. More fodder for the guilt I feel; don't blow it!!!

LOOKING BACK, BETH WAS MY FULFILMENT.

They say you are born with nothing, and you leave this earth with nothing… I don't believe that. True, you were born with nothing, and you will leave with no material possessions, even the clothes on your back; nevertheless, you leave behind, and with, memories. That is the one thing you bring to the afterlife.

I've had a good life… nay, a great life! A life I distinctly separated into three sections. The first stage was, of course, before I met Beth. That life was full of ignorance, stupidity, social ineptness; evolving through some form of self-realization, self-learning, and self-emulations; you have to learn somehow. Life was good, and yet, empty an unfulfilled.

Then I met Beth, and my world changed. Suddenly, there was responsibility in caring for another, two others actually, including George. I was not the centre of the universe anymore; family was my only focus. All I did from that time forward, was attempted to fulfill the needs and wants of the both of them. A home, food, financial stability, entertainment, activities, and most importantly, love, understanding, and guidance… leadership. I was raised up from a shell of a human into a functioning member of society. It is hard to understand how friends I had amassed before this time, were still with me… I was a real jerk!!

Then Nan came into my life, yes, from the time we got married, yet more significantly, from the time she moved in, and became a lasting fixture in our family unit. The nicest, most loving, and treasured person anyone could ever meet. With time came my daughter-in-law and two wonderful grandsons, and now with a sparkling enthusiastic grand daughter-in-law (hate that 'in-law' crap… they are all family, and I love them all).

My life was truly blessed.

And now… wow, what can I say? The rug has been pulled out from under me. Not totally of course, there are still friends, and parts of my loving family with me. This stage leaves me with a void. Loosing Nan, and Beth, combined with losing my parents, relatives, and friends, leaves me with the family, and friends, that I see far too rarely; not through any fault of their own, they have a life to live and to fulfill as I did. I'm not, nor do I want to be, on their doorstep, influencing their lives. I am lonely, grieving, and yet, what I have are memories to relive; memories that are waning as I age. I will leave this world loving and being loved, and I will bring memories to the afterlife with me. Not yet however, I have new memories to make and love to share in a new reality. Wish me luck!

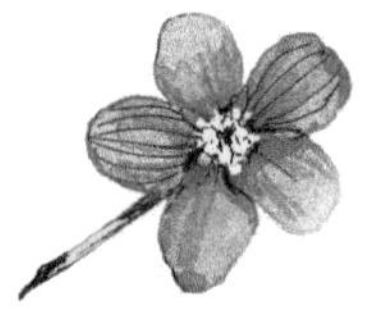

Chapter: In Closing

Life is not supposed to be pretty; otherwise, we would all be prince and princesses, living in 'La-La Land'!! It's what you do with your life that decides your fate!

OK, I lied!! Back on page one I said that my son, the journalist, would be the last person to review this book, and I was joking. He did get to review the quasi-finished product, and I'm glad he did. Turns out I didn't have to 'Capitalize' every second word, and I use way too many Exclamation Marks (see, I'm capitalizing again), and question marks as punctuations. The latter I ignored, as it reflects my vocal inflictive style of speaking. He also suggested a way to transform a 155 page 'self-help' book into the quasi-autobiography I was trying to effect; it is, after all, the story of a life altering experience during a traumatic part of my life. Love the finished product… Thanks Son!!!

There were many possibilities for a title for this book. It could have been 'Alzheimer's 101', or 'Alzheimer's for Dummies' (though that might have brought on a copywrite lawsuit or two). I thought of 'Alzheimer's, the last Frontier', or simply 'Oh Shit!' Realistically, I thought of 'Till Death Do Us Part'; however, I'm not dead yet, and I feel that somehow, spiritually, we have not yet parted. Her memory is still deep in my heart, and I feel Beth is still with me. Death is never the final answer, unless it is your own death, when you reunite for an eternity. She has passed away, and life is short; we'll be together again soon. Ahh, but I digress; I therefore determined a more appropriate title would be 'In Sickness and in Health'! I kept my vow, and I'm sure that no one will be mistaking to determine that this book is a plagiarism of a wedding ceremony.

Beth passed away three years ago, and though I was encouraged to write this book, I never felt I was ready; the journey was, and is still, not yet complete. So, what changed?? I chose this time to write because, with the onset, and the throws of what seems like an everlasting plague of COVID-19, I had a lot of time to reflect on my experiences, and the plague afforded me the time to write. Trust me when I say that it's not over yet, the experience I mean! The memories haunt me, and fits of grief, remorse, and guilt are being relived to the fullest as I write. Nightmares of losing Beth in a strange city bothers me immensely, and I realize I'm not there yet.

In the three years since Beth's passing, I felt the need to find distractions of sorts, to relieve the emptiness within, the pain of the treasured memories, the grief associated with those memories, and relinquish the guilt that so prevails. As the distractions kept me busy, I didn't have the time to write, and it seemed that moving on was desired, and yet inappropriate. If I got truly involved, the distractions might have become the 'new me', and the book might have never been started. I did meet some interesting acquaintances, none of which could compare with Beth. Don't get me wrong, the acquaintances I met were treasured and meaningful; however, not what I needed… nor lasting. I may find solace, and be at peace with moving on at some point in time; regardless, I will always have the love of Beth deep in my heart!

So how do I now feel about depression, grief, and guilt? "Been there, done that…again…and again…and again…" You must realize that writing this book was very emotional and traumatic for me… many times over!! Cathartic as it was, I had to relive a part of my life that, though I don't want to forget, I want to forget!

So why is it that every time I see a video with someone leaving a relationship… why is it every time I hear a song of a love lost, I still break out into tears?? It shows that I had a great love for Beth, and these instances bring back treasured memories, along with the sadness in the absence; and I'm ok with that.

Companionship!!! At seventy-four years of age, maybe I don't want to get into a lasting relationship…I haven't decided yet. I would like to find a companion of the opposite gender, male friends are easy to find; nevertheless, I would like to hold hands with someone, and get a few hugs in occasionally; not that there is anything wrong in having that form of relationship with the same gender…just not my preference. I feel very confident that I will flourish again, I must.

In summation, it appears I will not find love until I find peace, and I will not find peace until I find love! I do know; however, that this is but a temporary inconvenience. Have faith my friends! I feel that the love and peace we need will come to pass with the guidance of our dearly departed loved ones looking over our shoulders; it just takes patience.

This is the ending of this book, I have borne my soul, divulged my inner most feelings, rambled on incessantly about my love, grieving, and guilt, and yet it is not enough. Ending this book pains me deeply. It feels as if I must close this chapter in my life, leave this part of my life behind, and move on.

Though I know it will never truly end, I feel that this juncture is where I can no longer impart any further consolation, nor expectations; together we've been through it all, and I think that now is the time for the end of this story…

Still not ready!!

Written, in collaboration with J.Y.Lilly
Author of 'The Shard of History' series.
FreisenPress Publications.

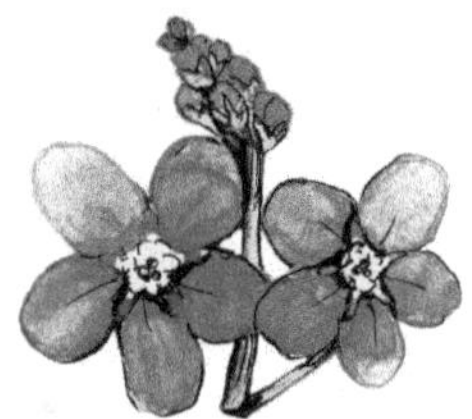

Addendum: Housekeeping

Disclaimer: The following was not researched, and is not intended to be taken as the gospel truth. It is a recollection of what occurred to me, and reflects a memory extending ten years previous. Also, bear in mind that the context of the content may vary based on which Province, State, Nation, Country, and even which political system you reside under. The intention is to simply invoke a thought process of the potential requirements pertaining to your specific situation. You must do your research!

There are a few items we need to get out of the way, specifically for your benefit. The first and foremost thing you must do, is to get your affairs in order… ASAP! I can't stress enough that Estate Planning is the most important thing you need to do.

This is a precautionary measure everyone should implement long before any tragedy befalls you, and/or your spouse; specifically, before diagnosis of a terminal disease, even more so, Alzheimer's. You must get a 'Last Will and Testament', '(Enduring) Power of Attorney' (POA), and a 'Personal Directive' prepared, and legalized, before your spouse is incapable of expressing her own desires, nor signing her name; with Alzheimer's, that occurs quickly. Once it's too late, you may not have the right to make any legal decisions on your loved one's behalf. Being a spouse is not always enough!!!

ESTATE PLANNING

A preliminary example of the importance of Estate Planning, is reference I made to Uncle Tom's passing on the first August, 2015. As it turned out, I rushed an online Last Will and Testament, got Uncle Tom to sign it, and had it witnessed by a head nurse at his facility… the next day he passed away, by surprise, before it could be notarized by a Notary Republic official.

As a result, the bank would not release the phenomenal amount of $1,500 he had in his account to cover expenses; I had no interest in his money and any remaining funds would go to his partner's next of kin. It turns out, he had not taken his partner, Maime, off as a joint account participant when she pre-deceased Uncle Tom 15 years prior. The bank would only release the fortune if I could provide a Death Certificate for Maime, and even then, I had to provide a Marriage Certificate for the two… I don't even think they were married, and they definitely had no children together.

I was finally able to make contact with Maime's daughter through a chance meeting at a London Drugs store about two months later. She was unaware Uncle Tom passed away. I filled her in on the situation and mentioned she could be the recipient of such a large inheritance, if she could produce a Marriage Certificate… she's probably still fighting the case.

GET YOUR AFFAIRS IN ORDER… **NOW**!!

PERSONAL DIRECTIVE

One of the decisions you must make, is regarding the Personal Directive for advanced, or end of life, health decisions should there be no reasonable expectation of recovery to an acceptable quality of life. This includes decisions regarding being kept alive by medications, artificial life-support, resuscitation, and intravenous feeding, amongst other procedures. It also includes the level of comfort care to be implemented, and what you determine as an acceptable quality of life to be.

This is a very personal choice that must not be taken lightly, and decisions that can only be made for yourself. You must think of the outcome of those decisions; do you want to be on life support when there is little chance of revival, or have resuscitation applied at all for that matter? This is pertinent to your spouse as well. I suggest you have a long and serious discussion with your spouse to determine her wishes while still able to do so.

It comes to mind that Personal Directives and POAs are made to protect yourselves from decisions made by anyone else, especially an abusive partner or relative. Your spouse's directive might be to keep her alive as long as possible, while you might instruct the acting physician to 'kick her to the curb'. Conversely, what your spouse's wishes are, might be private, and you have no right to become involved if it is against your spouse's wishes; if she wants it to remain between her and her lawyer, so be it. As such, it is very important to specify whom is to be awarded POA to invoke your choices.

Obviously, you are not yet invoking the POA or Personal Directive, just preparing them for the inevitable. To invoking a Directive, you will require a document from a doctor, identifying that your spouse is no longer capable of making her (or his) own decisions before a lawyer can invoke the POA and Directive.

When the time comes, and choices must be made on behalf of your partner regarding a level of care, or an end of life decision, the choice is never easily made. It is not a decision you will want to make at the last moment without knowing your spouse's wishes! It is a hard enough decision to make, even with everything in place, and knowledge of your spouse's wishes. Without knowledge of her wishes, the responsibility will fall on your shoulders, and the guilt will be yours to bear!!

More than 'care' or 'end of life' decisions, without these forms legalized, it will be difficult to release or sell anything. Anything you have registered, such as a joint bank accounts, property, cars, insurances, or any joint possessions, will have to be dealt with, even while your spouse is alive. Without a POA, this could include selling your house, your car, even simply resetting the pin code on her credit cards could be restricted, both before, and after her death. Be advised that invoking any of the above-mentioned changes, even with a death certificate, will be a burden; and that could be twenty years away.

These are just a few of the Estate planning issues that come to mind; nevertheless, use a lawyer, not an online form! There is no amount of money that is worth more! Don't cheap out on this! Being cheap now, will be your curse later. Heed my words, it will remove 90% of the stress you will experience through this journey. Trust me on this one!!

FINANCES

Finances are the next thing you should be aware of! When you are faced with the worst outcome in your life, finances will be the last thing you are thinking of; however, it could, and probably will bite you in the butt! One aspect you should consider, is whether you will have to sell your house and move closer to family or a care centre; that aspect cost us about $100K by not being prepared. If you are starting this journey, you might want to jump back to the chapter called 'The Necessity of Change', midway through this book.

You may not be aware that there are tax deductions you can claim regarding expenses related to the care of someone with such a disease. What you will need is a letter, from your doctor, indicating that there are medical issues that need additional attention, and expenses beyond normal life. You would be well advised to research what you are entitled to.

Medication is always in the forefront, yet medication is not the most expensive aspect of Alzheimer's. Additional expenses include medical assistance, homecare, respite costs, continuing care placement costs, wheelchairs, and the list goes on; even laundry for a patient in a care facility is an added expense.

There are also claimable visitation expenses, if your spouse is placed in a facility outside of your region (province or country specific). You might be tasked with driving vast distances for assessment and treatment in which food and mileage will be claimable for the both of you. Best to become informed of your allotment beforehand.

MISHAPS

Hate to be the bringer of bad news; nevertheless, there is another consideration you must be prepared for. Maybe 'prepare for' is the wrong terminology… more so, 'become aware of'! Of course, this involves both of you; nonetheless, potentially differently, and potentially resulting in a horrific situation; that my friend, are the calamities that could befall you if something unforeseen happens. I do cover more in relation to consequences of a mishap as it occurred to me, in the timeline, on February 1, 2015

The first aspect, of which I speak, is regarding your health and wellbeing! You may be male, you may be tough, you may be macho, yet none of those will protect you from breaking a leg or an arm… actually, any of those attributes will probably be the reason you do break your leg or an arm! Not a big deal you say? I couldn't agree more… if you were the only one of concern. Unfortunately, there is now someone in your care that won't agree.

So, the main consequence you must consider is what will happen to your spouse? At the onset of an Alzheimer's diagnosis, it may be a minor inconvenience if she is able to fend for herself, or for the both of you while you are hobbling around on crutches… she might even still be able to drive! What may not strike you right now is, what if you must stay in the hospital for an extended convalescence of a week, or even a month if your injury is more serious.

Conversely, her incarceration in a hospital must be considered pending an accident, or assessment of concern regarding her health and wellbeing; both physical and psychological. Based on the seriousness of her situation, she could be placed in a remotely located hospital, or at a specialized facility. Her staying in the hospital for an extended period of time will not be a cakewalk. In her confused state of mind, your sudden absence, and incapability to not be constantly by her side in a strange place will be devastating to her.

Moreover, and now comes the hammer, what if they determine she can't go home after the healing process? This could be because you are considered incapable of assisting her in a way that is required; your safety, or health is at stake and is a consideration; your home is not configured to the standard needed for her care requirements; or they determine her dementia has progressed to a point that she should not return home.

OK, now you are faced with a dilemma! She's in the hospital, and they say she can't go home. So what can you do? You might rationalize that now is the time for your spouse to be placed in a continuing care centre. That would be the obvious solution, besides, they are trained to take care of her… not so fast!! What preparation have you done to this point for her placement? So, you have things all lined up for placement, right?? Ah… think again; some have waited in the hospital for many months, even years before placement, even while on the waiting list… not a good situation at the best of times!

Be aware that they might tell you that you are on the hook to pay for her extended hospital stay; something you must be aware of, and prepared for! They don't care how they get their money, and some have even been advised that they could sell their home. Make sure this one concept is cleared up as soon as she is forced into prolonged hospital stay or it could bite you hard!!! If at all possible, it's a good idea to update your family health insurance before the diagnosis!

There is a vast difference between hospital care, and care in a long-term care facility! You don't get personalized care in a hospital; "Good morning! Should I book an appointment for the tennis court after your physiotherapy session or… oh wait, sorry, you can't get up; how silly of me??" "Would you like breakfast in bed this morning? Awe, just stay there, and we'll bring you lunch and dinner in bed as well!" While I'm incarcerated, I usually get the, "Get back in bed you idiot, doctor's orders!!" "You want what?" Of course, I'm making sarcastic fun of a serious situation; however, I'm trying to point out that hospitals are not necessarily the place you want someone you love to anguish in for months, and potentially years, even if they are mobile, and specifically with Alzheimer's.

PLACEMENT

Disregarding any casualty, disability, or any form of incarceration for either of you, there are different stages of dementia that must be considered with planned placement in a continuing care centre.

The first problem is that, at the onset of the disease, there is no way to identify when your spouse will require placement… her disease might last five years, maybe twenty. How far ahead should you place her on the placement waiting list? Short answer, no one knows, not even the doctor. I experienced times when I thought "This is it!!!", only to find that in a day or so she was fine for another week… or month… or more. There is no predefined schedule of degradation, as you will understand upon reading the timeline of events I went through.

My suggestion for you? Pray!!

CPSIA information can be obtained
at www.ICGtesting.com
Printed in the USA
BVHW060307150322
631484BV00005B/72